Raising Kids Who Choose Safety

Raising Kids Who Choose Safety

THE T.A.M.S. METHOD FOR CHILD ACCIDENT PREVENTION

DAVID C. SCHWEBEL, PhD

CHICAGO

Published by Parenting Press

An imprint of Chicago Review Press Incorporated

814 North Franklin Street

Chicago, Illinois 60610

ISBN 978-1-64160-792-6

Library of Congress Control Number: 2022935012

Cover design: Preston Pisellini

Typesetting: Nord Compo

Printed in the United States of America

Dedicated to the health and safety
of all children in our world

CONTENTS

ACKNOWLEDGMENTS

T HE JOURNEY OF WRITING A BOOK is unlike anything else I've done in life. The idealistic image of a solitary writer pecking away at a keyboard in some beautiful and inspirational locale—perhaps Hemingway's Key West or Thoreau's Walden Pond—has some bits of truth to it. But in reality, they are only small bits of truth.

Writing a book is truly a team effort. There might be one author who puts the words on paper, but there is a team behind that author. I thank my team.

For me, it starts with teachers and mentors. How does one learn to write, think, and convey ideas? I've had dozens of amazing teachers and mentors over the years, including especially Drs. Jerry Singer, Dorothy Singer, Niko Besnier, and Bill McGuire during my undergraduate years at Yale; Drs. Jodie Plumert and Jerry Suls during my graduate training at the University of Iowa; Dr. Matt Speltz during my clinical training at the University of Washington; and Drs. Jan Wallander, Michael Windle, Craig Ramey, and Sharon Ramey during my early years at the University of Alabama at Birmingham (UAB). I also learned to be a clinical psychologist from terrific supervisors in the clinics, including especially Drs. Dennis Harper at the University of Iowa and Chris McCurry at the University of Washington / Seattle Children's Hospital.

Learning to write, think, and convey ideas continues with one's own students. Over 150 students have trained in the UAB Youth Safety Lab, and I'm certain that I've learned as much from them as they have learned from me. Most continued on to successful careers themselves as child psychologists, mental health workers, physicians, and injury prevention specialists, and I thank each and every one of them for their contributions to the content of this book.

The detailed logistics of writing and publishing a book require lots of help as well. Thanks to Linda Konner, who served as my agent and supported me throughout the book-publishing journey. Thanks also to Michelle Williams and the terrific team at Parenting Press / Chicago Review Press for their guidance to transition a lengthy and bland Microsoft Word document into a beautiful book.

The children and families who inspired the vignettes in this book deserve recognition. No story you read is entirely true, but all are based on real-life situations. Many are based on real-life children I've known over the years. The children and families who inspired the stories will remain anonymous, but I greatly appreciate the inspiration they stimulated.

I also acknowledge the tremendous contributions from my friends and family. Life is short, and the special friendships I've developed at each stage of life will remain with me forever. An individual listing is not realistic, but one special shout-out goes to David Taylor and Lourdes Sánchez-López, who shared their own book-writing experiences and offered immense support during this voyage.

I come from a family of educators, psychologists, and book writers, and have fond memories of family vacations that involved writing. My grandparents Milton and Bernice Schwebel and Ruth Lubinsky, aunts and uncles Robert and Claudia Schwebel and Leonard and Marian Lubinsky, sister Sara Schwebel and sister-in-law Jiazhen Zhang, and especially my parents, Andrew and Carol Schwebel, each offered special guidance on writing, parenting, and educating children that shaped this book significantly. My niece and nephew, Miriam and Benjy Schwebel, the youth in our family, represent our future.

This book is about children, the future of our world. My wife, Yikun, and I raised our own children, Andy and Rosa, with delight. They are blossoming teenagers now. Through the TAMS (Teach, Act, Model, Shape) method—and much else—I know they have learned to keep themselves safe and to succeed in all that they do as they enter the independence of young adulthood. I thank Yikun, Andy, and Rosa for providing me the joys of parenthood and of seeing one's children grow up to be safe, smart, and successful.

I close with simple advice. Enjoy parenting. Take joy from the pleasures of seeing your children grow and successfully confront the challenges we all face. You will make a positive difference in your children's health and life by applying TAMS and creating a household culture of safety. This book will teach you how. Together we can help our children lead happy, healthy, and productive lives.

PART I

THE BASICS

1

ARE ACCIDENTS
REALLY A PROBLEM?

IF YOU'RE LIKE MOST PARENTS, you worry sometimes about your child's health. And you should. You visit the pediatrician for regular checkups. You seek vaccinations. You follow recommendations from your child's doctors and nurses.

You probably also think about your child's health from the perspective of safety. You have a car seat in your car—or a booster seat if your child is older—and you use it religiously. You may have installed devices such as cabinet locks and outlet covers if your children are young. If your children ride a bicycle, they wear bike helmets.

But do you really know all the risks? Let's consider a few surprising facts:

- Injury is the leading cause of death for everyone ages 1–44 in the United States and across much of the world.
- Among US children ages 1–14, injuries cause more deaths than the *next ten leading causes combined* (see following figure).

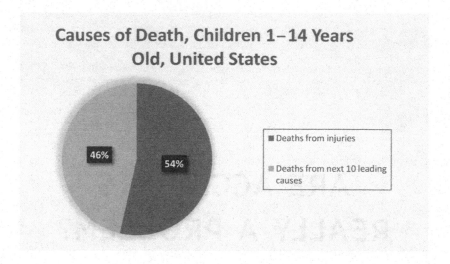

Causes of Death, Children 1–14 Years Old, United States

- Deaths from injuries
- Deaths from next 10 leading causes

46%　54%

- In the United States, over 11,000 children die from an injury every year. That's 30 children killed per day, more than one death every hour of every day.
- In the United States almost six million children visit an emergency department after an injury every year. That's about 16,000 injuries per day, 675 per hour, and over 11 serious child injuries every minute of every day of every year.

This book will reduce your risk of being one of those families.

Accidents Versus Injuries

We tend to think of injuries as "accidents," and that's accurate in some ways. We do not mean or intend for a child to get hurt. Kids do get hurt from time to time. After an injury, even a minor boo-boo, we parents feel bad. We sympathize with our child's pain and suffering.

However, you will learn from this book that most accidents can be prevented. Yes, accidents just happen—but you can prevent many and raise kids who choose safety.

In some cases prevention is simple. In other cases it is more complex. In all cases there are steps you can take to reduce the chances your child will be hurt or killed from an accident.

Let's consider a few examples. Here's Abigail's story:

I'm a new mom. I have a sweetheart baby boy, Tom, who just turned 20 months old. He's so cute! And he's so much fun! But he's also a handful sometimes. He just doesn't stop moving—walking and exploring and touching and tasting everything. Sometimes I feel like I can barely keep up with him.

The day after Tom's first birthday, my husband and I did a full makeover on our house. We put covers on all the outlets where Tom might play. We bought stair gates, and my husband got them installed on the top and bottom of the stairway. We put cabinet locks in the kitchen and bathroom, where we store cleaning supplies and medicines and other things like that. We even put padding on the edge of the fireplace hearth!

But last week the unthinkable occurred. We were really lucky it wasn't worse, but it sure gave me a major scare. Let me tell you what happened.

It was maybe around six thirty or seven on a Thursday evening. I was cleaning up the dishes in the kitchen. My husband was sitting on the sofa watching a football game. We were planning out the weekend—what shopping had to get done, what yardwork, and so on—and also when we might get a few hours together to ourselves. Baby Tom was in the living room playing. Both my husband and I could sort of see him if we peeked around the corner, and we could definitely hear him. That felt safe enough—he had a few toy trains and was pushing them around his model train tracks—he seemed to be quite content, and we were not worried. We had babyproofed the room, and we left him there like that all the time.

After a while I noticed that Tom was unusually quiet. My hands were covered with soap and dirty dishes, so I asked my husband to check what was going on. He peeked into the living room, and Tom was loading up his toy trains with pills! Yes—with medication pills! You see, every weekend,

I organize my weekly pills into a container so I don't forget to take them each day. I must have accidentally left the pills on the coffee table in the living room. Tom grabbed the container and was using my pills for cargo in his toy train. Can you believe it?

We asked Tom if he had eaten any, but I guess he was too young to give us a straight answer. It seemed he might have eaten some, so I started counting. Yup. I was pulling my pills out of his toy train, trying to find them all on the floor and in the little toy train cars! I wasn't positive, but it seemed that he might have eaten two of them—one of my birth-control pills and one Tylenol. We called the poison control center, and they said Tom would probably be fine if that was all he ate. But they suggested we take Tom to a doctor just in case, because Tylenol overdoses especially can be dangerous.

We went to the emergency room, and they ran a bunch of tests. In the end the doctor said the medicine would pass through Tom's system, and there didn't seem to be a major danger. We needed to keep an eye on him, and we should expect stomachaches and maybe some vomiting (sure enough, we had a late-night bed cleanup to deal with). Scary! We learned some good lessons. For sure, we need to watch Tom more carefully, *and* I need to always put my medications in a place Tom can't get them.

—Abigail, mom of Tom, age 20 months

Abigail and her husband learned a few key lessons. They need to put their medications—and anything else that might be dangerous to their young child—up and away, out of the child's reach. They learned the importance of supervising carefully. And they learned to expect the unexpected, like a toddler using pills for cargo in a toy train set.

In many cases the act of injury prevention isn't hard—putting medication away and supervising your child are really quite easy tasks in some ways. Remembering to do it always and consistently is much harder. We get busy and distracted and stressed, and it's easy to forget those easy things. Plus, anticipating possible problems and staying alert to safety concerns are challenges to all parents.

In this book we'll try to make the job a bit simpler. We'll outline simple steps you can take to improve your child's safety. Our goal together is to help you develop a culture of safety in your household so that safety lessons become second nature, safety precautions are expected, and your children stay injury free.

As Your Child Grows Older

Tom was just 20 months old and at a vulnerable age for injuries as he explored things around him in the house. Let's turn to April now, who is older, at age seven. By the elementary school years, safety concerns are somewhat different—but, as you'll see, our parental roles and responsibilities continue.

Spring has finally sprung! That means beautiful weather and time outdoors. In our family it's also birthday season—both of us parents have spring birthdays, as do our kids. This week was April's seventh birthday. Can't believe she is getting so old already.

One of April's favorite presents this year was a new set of Rollerblades. We were thinking she might enjoy using them around the neighborhood and also when we take her to the park. Seemed like a great idea at the time, but we clearly didn't think through all the issues surrounding kids and Rollerblades ahead of time.

You see, that first Saturday morning after her birthday, we were futzing around the house, and April was out in the yard. That's pretty common—we live in a safe neighborhood, and I didn't think much of it. But it turns out she was trying out her new Rollerblades in the driveway! Without us knowing about it.

The details are a bit sketchy, but it seems April was figuring out how to use the Rollerblades and somehow ended up in the street. Our driveway has a slight downhill slope toward the street, so that probably didn't help. Anyway she lands in the street and there's a car coming. The driver was a young guy—late teens / early 20s—and on his way to work at the shopping mall. I wonder if he might have been late to work and driving a little too fast—who knows? But that's not really the point.

So April is on her new Rollerblades and lands in the street. This young guy is driving by, sees April, and swerves away to miss her. He avoids April but crashes into a car parked across the street. We heard the crash and looked out the window. We could see what had happened. April was sitting in the road crying. The young man jumped out of his car and went to April. Thankfully he just picked her up and put her on the grass in the neighbor's yard. He was smart to get her out of the road in case another car came by. At that point, of course, we ran outside to help April and to talk to the young man.

Eventually the police came by and wrote up a report. We'll have to deal with the insurance companies and costs and all, but more important we have to deal with the safety issues with April. How could all this have happened? My husband and I sat down that night and listed out things that needed to change immediately. First, three rules for April:

- April should never use her Rollerblades without an adult supervising her.
- April should never use her Rollerblades (or any other outdoor toy) at the bottom of the driveway near the street, even if an adult is directly supervising her.
- April should always wear a helmet and kneepads when Rollerblading (we agreed the kneepads might not be needed as she gets older and more experienced, but for now she needs them).

And two rules for us:

- We should play outside more often with April and supervise her in activities she enjoys but might be dangerous, such as Rollerblading.

> - We should always ask April what she is going to do before she goes outside to play when we are not going outside with her.
>   —Pat and Jim, parents of April, age seven

Pat and Jim were exactly right. By age seven, children can start to learn and follow rules. That improves safety. But there are other lessons here too. Pat and Jim's rules will help April learn to practice safety and will likely generalize to other situations. That helps them create a culture of safety in their home. And that culture will be manifested: April will learn to wear safety gear (helmets) and to stay away from risks (play at the top of the driveway, away from traffic).

Pat and Jim learned some lessons for themselves too. Parenting responsibilities continue throughout childhood. We need to supervise, both directly (go outside and interact with April when possible) and indirectly (when you can't go outside with her, ask what your child is going to be doing and periodically check to be sure she is still safely doing what she planned).

It's not always easy. We lead busy lives, and our children always seem to find risks we don't anticipate. But there are plenty of steps we can take to improve safety, and every incremental step will create a safer household and safer children. That's our goal—incremental steps to inch purposefully toward reducing the risk of an accident through a household culture of safety.

Aren't Some Kids Just "Accident Prone"?

You may be thinking to yourself something along these lines: *I can't stop my kid from getting hurt. It just happens. He's clumsy. She's careless. I was always getting hurt as a kid. It's not surprising that my own kids would be like me.*

To some extent you're right. Some children are clumsier than others, and some children are more careless than others. One research study after another has demonstrated that one of the best predictors of a child getting hurt is if the child got hurt before. So yes, some children are more "accident prone" than others.

But that doesn't mean you can't take steps as a parent to change those patterns. We'll discuss those ways as we move forward, but first let's address the issues of clumsiness and carelessness.

Several years ago I worked with some colleagues on a big research study examining clumsiness and accident risk. We asked children to complete basic tests of clumsiness. Could they throw and catch balls successfully? Could they balance on one foot? On a balance beam? Could they pour water from one container to another without spilling it? Could they quickly string beads onto a piece of yarn? We put all those measures together to get a clumsiness score for each child. And then we compared their clumsiness scores to their injury histories.

Guess what? There was nothing there. Clumsy children didn't get hurt any more often than nonclumsy children. Their injury rates were about equal. One explanation for the result is that clumsy children know they are clumsy, and so they avoid taking risks. Agile children think they're physically skilled, so they take more risks—and sometimes get hurt.

As to carelessness, we know all children are a bit careless. Their brains are not developed yet to adult levels, so kids are forgetful, impulsive, and messy. They don't always know what is safe or dangerous, and they fail to think about the consequences of their actions. It's likely that some children act these ways more than others, and that may lead some kids to get hurt more often than others.

Should we parents just give up, then? Should we Bubble-Wrap our children with protective gear and confine them with excessive safety rules to keep them safe and avoid injury risk at all costs?

No, and no.

Children need to try new things. They need to explore the world. They need to jump and climb and taste and dig. That's how they grow and learn and understand.

Our goal in this book is not to Bubble-Wrap our children to keep them from doing anything that might be dangerous. In fact, quite the opposite. We want children to learn and explore and try new things. Yes, older children should wear helmets on their bikes and shin guards on the soccer field. Younger children should live in homes where the pills are placed in containers with child-resistant lids and the cleaning supplies are placed into cabinets with cabinet locks. Some protection—yes, even a touch of Bubble Wrap—is sensible and logical. Too much is suffocating.

The challenge—amid the many other challenges of parenting—is to find the right balance. We want our children to grow and explore, but we want them to do so safely. We might accept a few cuts and bruises along the way, but no parent should be ready to accept broken bones, concussions, or near-fatal injuries as "part of growing up." In this book we'll discuss how you can work with your family to discover the right balance so your children grow up in a safe and healthy way.

Isn't This Just the Reality of Today's World?

You may be thinking to yourself: *Of course my kid takes risks. He's just copying what he sees in his video games.* Or you may be thinking, *Well, look at what the superheroes do—Wonder Woman flies, so my daughter tries to fly. Spiderman climbs, so my son climbs. Usually it's fine, but sometimes silly mistakes happen, and that leads to occasional bumps and bruises.*

In some ways you're right. Most of today's children are exposed to immense amounts of media. They scroll through YouTube endlessly. They chat addictively on social media. They play video games on phones and tablets, watch movies constantly, and even occasionally catch a glimpse of old-fashioned cable television.

All this media exposure leads children to mimic the heroes they see in the media. They emulate superheroes with superhuman speed and power and the ability to fly, who never get hurt. They admire social media influencers who engage in ridiculous and sometimes downright dangerous activities online. They play video games showing unrealistic scenes, and they mindlessly stream material designed for much older audiences.

Without a doubt all this media exposure impacts young and growing minds. In fact, research in my lab found that frequent exposure to superhero media may cause children to take risks when they are unsupervised and given an opportunity. We also found that popular children's movies frequently include scenes with risky behaviors such as driving without seat belts or crossing streets recklessly. And we know that children observe these details, learn from them, and copy them.

What's a parent to do? Just like we can't Bubble-Wrap our children to prevent injury, we also can't fully remove them from today's world of media influences. It's just not realistic, at least in my family. Instead I recommend three strategies.

First, do what you can to moderate the influence of media by helping your child choose age-appropriate entertainment that leans toward safe and smart behaviors. This isn't easy, but you as a parent can guide your children and their media choices. You'll learn more about shaping as you read on in this book, and shaping is an excellent way to help your child find media that leads to safer behaviors.

Second, we must choose our own media sources wisely. Think about times when your child is present and you have the television on in the same room. What are you watching, and what might your child pick up on occasionally? Is there dangerous or unrealistic risk-taking on the show? Does your child catch glimpses of those scenes and take note? We'll talk more about modeling as we move forward in the next few chapters. Modeling safe choices yourself will lead your child to make safe choices.

Third, we can supervise. You'll learn more about this sort of action, too, as you read on in the book. Even if your toddler does want to try to fly like Superman, if you are supervising him carefully as he prepares his launchpad on the living room sofa, you can intervene and guide him to a safer option. Similarly, if your fourth-grader wants to jump her dirt bike over a homemade ramp in the backyard like her favorite YouTuber, your supervision can redirect her to a safer activity.

In short, we parents have power. Not the power of superheroes but the power to shape and influence our children's behaviors. Our children live in dangerous worlds, and we can and should let them explore those worlds. They need to see things and touch things and climb things and yes, even jump off things in order to grow up. We have the power to allow and encourage those activities.

At the same time, we parents have a lot more wisdom and experience and thinking skills than our children do. There are times when we need to watch them, teach them, restrict them, and help them. This book will help you determine how and when to take those actions, and ultimately how to create an overarching culture of safety in your household that reduces your children's risk of injury.

2

CREATING A CULTURE OF SAFETY

MANY PEOPLE SAY, "Accidents happen." Indeed, they happen with disturbing frequency. Accidents are the leading cause of child death in the United States and much of the world.

Accidents are preventable. If something different had occurred—if children did something different, adults did something different, or the environment were different—then most accidents would not happen. Our goal as parents must be to increase the frequency of those different events. We can create a culture of safety in our homes that will interrupt pathways to an injury event.

Luckily, we get help. Parents lead the way in many cases, but plenty of other people are invested in our children's safety as well. Government bodies regulate to reduce injury risk. Other adults in our children's world, such as their teachers, babysitters, lifeguards, and police officers, help reduce injury risk. And through our parenting, children also help themselves. If we can teach and shape children to behave safely, they will make wise decisions to keep themselves safe.

A Model of Injury Risk

In most cases injuries are not caused by any single factor. Instead a wide range of factors come together to create risk. This situation creates mixed news. On the negative side, it means that it is hard to generalize from one injury to another. When our child gets the flu, we learn we should get a flu vaccine next year to avoid a recurrence. But when our child gets a broken arm, we don't really have a clear pathway to prevent the next time. In fact, there are a load of child injury prevention strategies, and combined they are likely to reduce risk but not necessarily prevent all negative outcomes.

The following figure illustrates some of the factors that contribute to particular injury events, and this leads us to think about a really positive aspect of the complexity of injuries and injury prevention.

Look at the figure carefully. You'll see that there are many different factors that come together to create an injury situation at the

Factors That Influence Child Injury Risk

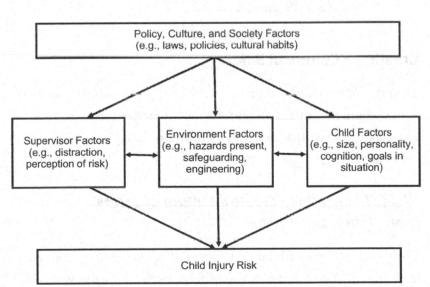

bottom of the figure. The child's personality, cognitive (thinking) skills, physical size and strength, and social patterns contribute. So does the adult supervisor—what are her habits and what is she doing in the situation? Of course, the environment makes a difference—what risks are present? And then there are bigger issues, such as government policies, culture, and the weather. It's all quite complicated!

Here's the good news: if you can create a culture of safety and prevent any single aspect of the many factors that merge together to produce a child's injury, you will prevent that injury. That's right—you don't have to disrupt *all* those arrows in the figure, you only have to stop *one* of them to prevent the injury from occurring. Imagine your child is playing in a risky way on a dangerous playground. He is climbing up a metal jungle gym and ready to jump from the top down to a concrete pad, pretending to be Superman. Despite the risk-taking behavior of your child and the risky environment he is playing in, if you are supervising carefully, you can step in and intervene before your child jumps. A single blocked pathway—achieved in this case through careful supervision—will avert the injury, allowing your Superman to reach the ground safely.

Creating a Culture of Safety

Throughout this book we'll return to the theme of a culture of safety. A household that thinks about safety will practice safety. So how do you create a home that practices a culture of safety? Good question. Let's run through a quick Q&A.

What Should I Do to Create a Culture of Safety in My House, and When?

This book offers many ideas. Chapter 3 covers most of the basic information. You'll learn to follow four steps: (1) teach your child about safety, (2) act to supervise and safeguard your home, (3) model safe behaviors, and (4) shape your child within a household culture of safety. We call this the TAMS method: teach, act, model, and shape.

How Will I Know When I Am Succeeding?

This is a tough one because the answer might be disappointing: you won't know. Scientists describe injuries as a low base-rate event, which means they happen frequently to the whole population of all children. But each individual child may go several days, weeks, or even months before they experience a minor injury. Some children will have major injuries every now and then, but some children may never experience a serious injury at all. So if you prevent your child from getting hurt, you may not even realize it because the injuries happen so infrequently. You'll be making an infrequent event for your child even more infrequent, and the change may be impercep tible to you.

Plus, to be honest, even if you follow all the advice in this book, your child may still get hurt occasionally. Our goal is to reduce risk. Having a goal to entirely remove risk just isn't realistic.

It's not all bad news here, though. You likely can detect a change in your household's culture. By creating a culture of safety in your home, you, your partner, your children, and everyone else in your home will be thinking about safety in a different way. Safe engage-ment will come to your mind as you take on your daily activities. You will store your scissors away from your toddler, keep a close eye on your fourth-grader as he learns to boil spaghetti on the stovetop, or double-check that you have the right car seat for your child's age and size. The changes might not be bluntly obvious, but if you are observant (or if you blog, jot down notes, or take relevant pictures occasionally), you will sense some changes as they occur.

In some cases, you'll even be able to quantify change. Does everyone in the house wear their seat belt, always, every time they are in the car? Do you check your smoke detectors a few times each year? Are your medications and cleaning supplies always stored in a safe location, away from young children? Our goal is for these things to become second nature—you do them automatically and without thinking. In fact, many of us may already meet some of these goals—for example, we might always wear our seat belts. Expanding to other safety domains will quickly create a culture of safety in your house that is then adopted as normal for your children.

What Should I Do Differently Next Time If My Child Does Get Hurt?

The short answer is that it depends on the circumstances of the injury. No matter what, you are likely to learn one or more lessons. Reflect on the circumstances of the injury and the various pathways that led to it. Use the figure in this chapter to guide your thinking. Perhaps you could do something different to prevent the next time by blocking one or more pathways of causality—safeguard your home, supervise more carefully, or place risky objects in a safer place. But perhaps someone else has to do something different—your partner, your child's school, or your government's policymakers. And perhaps you need to teach your child new rules (and then ensure she follows them), or train your child to think or act differently. Most likely several of these things might make sense, but that will vary widely across the circumstances of the injury that occurred. A parent who practices a culture of safety will review injury events, ponder them, and then make changes appropriate to the situation.

Let's consider a story from Jonah, the father of three boys:

Wow, what a Saturday it's been! Not unusual for a house with three boys, I guess. But this was a really terrible Saturday for our family. It's painful to even tell the story.

I was out at Aaron's soccer game—he's our oldest boy, age eight. My wife was with baby Adam. He's just three months old, and my wife was doing the usual baby stuff with him, feeding and rocking to sleep and diaper changes, whatever. Abraham is the middle boy. He's four years old now—almost five—and I guess he kind of fits the middle child syndrome.

Abraham was in the playroom and discovered Aaron's toy airplane. This is a battery-operated, remote-control thing—you push some buttons and the airplane kind of flies around. It's supposed to be for older kids—the label says AGES 12 AND UP, so I'm not even sure why Aaron has it, but it's certainly not a good toy for a four-year-old like Abraham to discover.

So apparently Abraham finds this toy and starts playing with it. Amazingly he was smart enough to take it outside in the backyard—and he starts flying the airplane around. All of a sudden, my wife hears a loud shriek and yelling and crying. She runs out to the backyard and discovers Abraham holding his face and sobbing. The airplane and remote control are lying on the grass.

I'll leave out the horrible, gory details, but several hours later it became clear to us that Abraham had a very serious eye injury. The airplane somehow flew straight into his right eye. And this is where it gets really bad. The doctors say he may never have vision in that eye again. I can't believe it. He definitely will never have completely normal vision in the eye. There is hope he might recover some sight, but even that is uncertain.

It just doesn't seem possible. Abraham is only four years old, and the vision in his right eye is damaged forever. We have good genes for longevity on both sides of our family, so he might live to be in his 80s or even his 90s. That's 75 or more years of living with bad vision or possibly blindness in his right eye. Just because he flew a toy airplane in the backyard on a sunny Saturday afternoon. I'm having trouble accepting it still.

Well anyway, what lessons have we learned? An awful lot. Let me see if I can summarize where everything went wrong:

- Abraham should have known not to play with his older brother Aaron's toys. We've told him that before, but he seems to ignore those rules a lot.

- Aaron should have stored his toy in his bedroom or on a high shelf, or somewhere Abraham couldn't access it. We've told him that too, but again the kids don't always follow the rules. Probably my wife and I need to do a better job of monitoring where toys are stored and make sure Aaron's toys are kept separate from Abraham's. And this will get even more complicated when Adam gets a little older.

- My wife and I should never have had the airplane in the home in the first place. It was designed for children ages 12 and up, and our oldest son is only eight. I have to admit I sometimes ignore those rules—they seem kind of silly to me. So probably I bought the airplane for Aaron's Christmas present. I'll take the blame on that one—hard lesson learned.

- My wife should have been supervising Abraham more closely. I know she was busy with baby Adam, but somehow we need to learn to watch two kids at once. Abraham is still young, and we really can't trust him to stay safe on his own.

- Not sure on this one, but perhaps there should be more safeguards on the airplane toy. Abraham is only four, but it seems like an older child or even an adult might do the same thing—fly the airplane into your face and eye. It's a dangerous toy. Should it be allowed? Or should you have to wear safety goggles if you operate it? Whose fault is that? Not sure—maybe government regulators? Or the company that made the toy airplane?

—Jonah, dad of Aaron, age eight,
Abraham, age four, and Adam, age three months

Jonah and his wife learned quite a bit here, didn't they? Abraham's life—and really all their lives—will never be the same.

The injury was caused by the unfortunate circumstance of many things coming together, including the purchase of a toy inappropriate for the children in the home, the storage of the toy in a location accessible to a young child, and the poor supervision of that child. There also are questions about the safety of the toy and whether government policies or the manufacturer might have designed it with better safeguards. And there were environmental factors: Abraham's ability to access the backyard unsupervised and perhaps even issues like the wind blowing in the yard that day.

What lessons can Jonah and his wife—and you—learn? Jonah outlined some of the lessons for us, any one of which might have prevented the serious eye injury. I agree with Jonah's list, and it illustrates beautifully that there are many pathways to prevent an injury. It also shows how you can enact several strategies simultaneously to reduce the risks of injury and create a culture of safety in your home.

3

SO WHAT SHOULD I DO?
THE TAMS METHOD

WE'VE ESTABLISHED THAT ACCIDENTS occur because many factors come together at the right time and place. We've also established that interrupting any one of those pathways can prevent an accident. And we've established that creating a culture of safety in your household will help you block those paths, making your home a safer place for your children and allowing you to raise kids who choose safety.

It's important to recognize that you are not entirely alone in your desire to keep your children safe. In fact, most everyone in society desires injury-free children. We know that government policymakers look out for our children, passing all sorts of regulations and requirements to make our children safer. We also know that various people in the spheres of our children's lives—teachers, religious leaders, lifeguards, police officers, physicians, nurses, and many others—help to protect our children. But ultimately we are the parents, and we have responsibility to safeguard our children.

Great, so how do we do it? All parents want to keep their children safe. Creating a culture of safety in your home probably sounds like a good idea. You probably know to put your toddler in a car seat and give your 10-year-old a bicycle helmet. But what else? Can you actually prevent your child from getting hurt?

Some parents seem to think injuries just happen—they are the result of bad luck, fate, or destiny. They just occur, it's part of kids growing up, and parents really shouldn't bother trying to prevent them. Some parents even think injuries are good for their children—an accident teaches the child a good lesson or helps them grow up.

Of course, these beliefs are incorrect. Parents truly can help prevent their children's injuries. In fact, parents can do a tremendous amount to create a culture of safety and reduce their children's risk of accidental injuries. Your parenting contributions fit into four categories: teach, act, model, and shape, or TAMS.

THE TAMS METHOD

Teach
Act
Model
Shape

Teach

Some of us enjoy teaching, and others less so. Whether we enjoy it or not, parenting always involves **teaching**. For those who don't really like to teach, it helps to remember that parenting is a lot different from our standard prototype of what teaching might involve. In parenting there are no classrooms, no desks, and no textbooks. Lectures are rare and chalkboards nonexistent. The teaching of parenting happens in short bursts, at opportune moments, and with whatever tools happen to be present at the time. Consider this example from Ashley:

I was on the way home from picking up Amelia, my four-year-old, from preschool. I needed to stop by the supermarket to grab a few items for dinner. The market was crowded, so we had to park quite a long way from the front door. I got out of the car and unbuckled Amelia from her car seat. A lot was on my mind—problems at work, figuring out what to put on the dinner table, and whether I could squeeze out another day without doing the laundry at home. I took Amelia's hand, and we started to walk toward the market.

Then I remembered TAMS—here was an opportunity to teach. We were just walking across the parking lot, and my mind was racing about the problems of the day. I could've just held Amelia's hand and gotten her safely into the market. But I noticed a car starting to back up. I stopped. And thanks to the *T* in TAMS, I said to Amelia, "Did you notice that car backing up? The little white lights were shining, which means it was driving backward. We have to be careful when walking in a parking lot." Simple, huh?

Then as we approached a parking lot thoroughfare, I said to Amelia, "Let's look both ways for traffic and make sure the cars are stopped before we cross into the market." She didn't become a safe pedestrian in a day, that's for sure. She's only four years old, after all. But perhaps she learned a bit of a lesson, and I can remind her next time I take her to the market. I was glad I could put aside my daily worries to practice TAMS. It was a great opportunity to teach Amelia something about crossing parking lots safely.

—Ashley, mom of Amelia, age four

Ashley found a great opportunity to teach her child about safety. It was quick and easy, and it certainly taught Amelia a lesson. For some rare parents, such opportunities are grasped naturally. Those parents will not just say to their two-year-old, "Look at the car," but rather, "Look at the red car"—a subtle and easy way to teach their child about colors.

Other parents—most of us—need to teach ourselves to use such strategies. It takes a little work, but it's not hard. Whenever you are with your child, look for opportunities to interact and engage. And while you interact and engage, look for opportunities to teach your child something you know and they don't (and yes, there is plenty that you know and they don't, even when they grow to be teenagers).

Some of those lessons will be about safety—how to decide what to do and what not to do in places where there might be danger. You cross streets, step onto escalators, walk around icy spots on the sidewalk, boil water, and use scissors quite automatically. But your child needs to learn. You can teach during the daily activities of life just by explaining what you are doing and why you are doing it that way.

Teaching safety is the first step of TAMS, and it will help you make your family safer, healthier, and happier. But teaching is only the first step. You also need to *act* for safety.

Act

One of the great long-term joys of parenthood is seeing your child grow from a small baby to a young adult and beyond. We notice most obviously the physical growth—replacing outgrown clothes, shopping for new shoes, and the tricky first purchases of deodorant, bras, and razors.

But along with that physical growth comes mental growth. Children learn to act in safer ways. Before they learn, as they learn, and even sometimes after they've learned, a parent's actions protect their children. That's what the *A* in TAMS is for: the adult's **actions**.

We can divide actions into two subcategories: supervision and safeguarding. To understand the distinction, let's consider a social science concept: active versus passive interventions.

We all know what an intervention is—something that is meant to block something else from happening. So politicians might intervene to prevent wars, therapists might intervene to prevent a divorce, and attorneys might intervene to prevent an execution. When it comes to safety, we are intervening to prevent an accident: we try to do something to prevent an accident from occurring.

Social scientists place interventions on a continuum ranging from active to passive. Fully active interventions require someone to actively complete something to prevent the accident. As an example, lifeguards are a form of active intervention. They are hired with the primary task of taking action to prevent drownings.

Passive interventions, on the other hand, are put in place to prevent accidents without any activity from a person. An example of a passive intervention is a guardrail at the side of the highway. Once that guardrail is installed, it will reduce the severity of an accident by preventing a vehicle from tumbling off a cliff and injuring the passengers inside.

The distinction between active and passive intervention is not a dichotomy but a continuum. Most interventions fall somewhere along that continuum. They have some degree of active intervention and some degree of passive intervention.

Why does all this social science matter? Because your actions as a parent can comprise *both* active and passive interventions. In fact, to keep your child safe, you will need to engage in both types of interventions.

In many ways more-passive interventions are easier. Once you do something, it's done. You can engage in passive interventions by safeguarding your child's environment. You are probably familiar with some simple strategies: place plastic covers on electrical outlets where your toddler may play, connect and test smoke and carbon monoxide detectors in your home, and install cabinet locks to restrict your child's access to dangerous cleaning supplies in the cupboards. In fact, the list of passive interventions you might enact is substantial, and we will describe many of them as you read on.

The hardest part of passive interventions—those interventions that safeguard your child's environment with some degree of permanency—is taking the first step. Once you get a stair gate installed, it will be there. Once you get a locking cabinet to store your firearms, they will be safer. Schedule these tasks in your calendar. Order devices online, and install them as soon as they arrive. In short, be your own taskmaster. Give yourself a deadline and just get the tasks done. Force yourself to take these easy steps of mostly passive interventions, and avoid tragedy by accomplishing simple tasks.

More complicated are the tasks that require active intervention. These tasks generally revolve around supervision—you need to watch your children to keep them safe.

There's no getting around it: diligent supervision is really hard. It can be repetitive, tiresome, and even sometimes boring. Averting your eyes for even just a few moments can be tragic if your child discovers items that are sharp, poisonous, hot, or otherwise dangerous. And averting your eyes is so tempting when you've got a smartphone full of social media in your hands—plus a kitchen needing cleaning, clothes needing ironing, and a dog needing walking.

How to balance it all? There are no magical solutions, but just remember that safety and security must come first. If there is risk to your child where she is, you must protect her. If you can place her in a safe playpen, or as she gets older a safe room, you might be able to reduce the intensity and proximity of your supervision—you can be a little laxer. But only if your child is in a safe place, away from danger.

Of course, as children grow older, your supervision can also become laxer. But take those steps slowly. Merge your passive interventions to create a safe environment with your relaxing of active supervision as children mature. Find the right balance, always tilting toward safety when in doubt.

Model

Classic research in the injury prevention field sought to figure out what factor best predicted teenagers' use of seat belts when they drove a car. Would it be their gender? Did girls wear seat belts more than boys? Perhaps it would be their age or their driving experience: Would older or more-experienced drivers wear seat belts more often? Or perhaps it would be their driving habits: Would teens who drive more often, at faster speeds, or for longer distances wear their seat belts more often?

All of those factors played a role, but none of them was the best predictor of whether the teens would wear a seat belt. The actual most influential factor? Their parents' seat-belt use. That's right. If you, as a parent, use your seat belt, your child is likely to do so also. That's more important than your child's gender, age, experience, driving habits, or almost anything else.

At all ages, including the teenage years and beyond, our children learn from watching us. Whether you like it or not, and whether you know it or not, your actions carry a lot of weight. If you **model** safety, your child will learn to act safely. If you model taking a lot of risks, I'm afraid your child will be likely to take risks.

So think about what you do, especially when your children are present. Use your seat belt while driving or flying, of course. But also use your helmet while biking or skiing, your life jacket while boating or fishing, and your protective eyewear while woodworking or Weedwacking.

Think also about other risky behaviors. Do you text while you drive? Leave pot handles facing outward while cooking? Speed when you're late? Do your children notice, absorb, and ultimately emulate these behaviors?

Reversing long-term habits is hard. Take a look at LaToya's story to see how one mom managed to accomplish it.

I've always been a jogger. My morning runs keep me physically healthy and also mentally healthy. Without them I feel lost. Every morning I get out of bed, down a quick cup of coffee, and set off for two, three, or even five miles sometimes. Earbuds are in, blasting my favorite tunes, and I just hit the pavement. Doesn't matter if it's cold or hot or rainy or sunny, I need that run. The music really helps me feel good too. I'll admit, I blast it—really loud. Just keeps me going. Been doing it the same way for years and years.

Now that Junior is playing middle school soccer, he goes out for runs too. I love seeing him set out. Occasionally we go together, but to be honest, I can't keep up with him. Hate to admit it, but his 12-year-old legs and lungs are stronger than mine. And he likes to run later in the day—not an early bird like me.

So one afternoon, Junior was setting off to run and I saw him put his music on. Wow, was it loud! I could hear music from his earbuds all the way across the living room. How could he possibly hear traffic? I know how scary it is sometimes to run on the roads and see cars zipping by. You need to be able to hear the cars coming to keep safe. Not to mention the damage he's probably doing to his young ears. I've read that loud music can slowly cause damage to your hearing, and you might become deaf in old age. I don't want that to happen to him.

Then—oh my gosh—it hit me! Junior was just listening to music the same way I do. I blast my music when I run, and he surely knew that—he sometimes sees me getting ready in the morning and blasting the music when I leave, and also when I get back home. Like mother, like son. What will happen to my hearing as I age? And am I hearing the traffic on the roads? What have I done?

I set out to make changes right away. I talked to Junior and admitted my mistake. That was hard to do—to tell your 12-year-old that you were doing something wrong. But I needed to do it. He listened, and I think he heard me. From then on, I turned my music down—*way* down. I still enjoy my run every day, and I still listen to music. But I can also hear the traffic now. And I can even hear the birds chirping and the kids playing in yards as I run past. What a delight! I'm probably saving my hearing for the future too.

Junior listened. He runs for soccer training still, but he has his music turned down like he should—at least when he leaves the house. No, seriously, I trust him, and I think he leaves the music turned down for the full run. He's a good kid and he respects me, and I think we both learned a valuable lesson on this one.

—LaToya, mom of Junior, age 12

LaToya's lesson was a hard one, but it illustrates the power of change. She changed herself, and her 12-year-old son followed. It took guts. It also took a tough conversation to admit fault to her son. But in the end, she and Junior protected their safety—and their hearing.

Shape

The final letter in TAMS refers to **shape**. Shaping is helping your children learn about safety as they grow older. This is probably the hardest of the four TAMS pieces to accomplish. It takes time and practice. But it's also critical because it represents the foundation of a household's culture of safety.

What exactly are you shaping? Stated simply, your child's ability to learn, understand, and follow rules. Why is it hard? Because children have the natural proclivity to explore, push limits, and try new things. This proclivity to explore is generally healthy. It helps them learn about the world. It helps them grow and mature. But it also can lead sometimes into habits of disregarding rules that are hard to break.

Whole books—lots of them, in fact—have been written about how parents can shape their children to heed rules. In general the principles are the same:

- Parents must be consistent. There are no special circumstances when rules can be broken.
- Parents must be firm. When a rule is violated, the child is stopped and disciplined. The discipline may be a simple verbal warning but should be issued nonetheless.
- Positive behavior should be rewarded. This is really important. Parents should praise children when they do follow the rules. In fact, praising rule-following will be much more powerful to shape behavior than punishing rule-breaking.

So that's the deal. Set rules and enforce them consistently. Praise and reward your child when she does the right thing. Do this a lot. Stop your child when she does something wrong, caution and remind her what would be a safer choice, and move on. Don't lavish positive or negative attention for rule violations—children tend to like the attention and will repeat their behavior to obtain more of it. A downward spiral will quickly emerge if parents spend most of their time disciplining and redirecting their children away from negative activities rather than engaging and teaching them through positive ones. Instead lavish attention for doing things right and following the rules. Spend time with your children (part of the teach and act in TAMS), and enjoy that time.

The Power of TAMS: Teach, Act, Model, Shape

You have the power to prevent tragic injuries in your household. The TAMS method offers the pathway to that goal.

Many aspects of TAMS are easy. You can easily *teach* your child at opportune moments, just like Ashley recognized she could teach her daughter about pedestrian safety in the supermarket parking lot. You can also *model* safe behaviors—Ashley didn't mention it, but she was not texting as she walked across the parking lot, and this is a good thing. Distracted pedestrian behavior is dangerous, just like distracted driving, and TAMS guides us on the strong influence of modeling.

Many parts of the *acting* portion of TAMS are also easy to implement. Steps such as moving cleaning products to higher shelves, installing outlet covers, and checking your smoke detector take less than a minute. Installing car seats, cabinet locks, and stair gates are a bit more involved but still quite manageable. The less passive and more active interventions involved in the acting portion of the TAMS method are harder. Supervision of young children takes patience, perseverance, and diligence. But active supervision is achievable, and it saves lives.

The last component of TAMS is *shaping*, and this is also the hardest. Working to shape your children's behavior so they learn, remember, and follow rules is a long-term process. But it yields a lifetime of health, happiness, and safety, so it's well worth the effort. Follow the simple principles of enforcing consistent rules, firmly stopping behavior that disregards rules, and amply and consistently rewarding positive behavior, and you'll be well on your way to creating a safe environment for you and your children.

I'll make one last point about TAMS before we start thinking about specific strategies and techniques you can use to reduce injury risk in your household. Everything you do to follow the TAMS method must be couched in thinking about your child's age and ability. To state the obvious, you would never teach a two-year-old the complexity of climbing playground equipment the way roofers are taught to climb ladders (three points always on the ladder: two hands and one foot or two feet and one hand). Nor would you teach a 10-year-old basic safety guidelines such as "don't run with scissors." They already know such rules.

Most decisions about how to apply TAMS based on a child's age are much subtler, however. Children develop in interesting ways. You know your child best, and you probably know what he can and can't handle. Carefully consider your child's age and ability to judge what he can and can't absorb, learn, and act upon for safety.

PART II

SAFETY AS CHILDREN GROW

4

INFANCY

Ages 0–11 Months

EW EVENTS CHANGE ONE'S LIFE more than having a baby. The emotions are a roller coaster—joy, love, and happiness, to be sure, but also exhaustion, confusion, uncertainty, and feelings of being overwhelmed. Depression and sadness can also emerge, and simple household chaos is common.

As parents experience these myriad emotions and feelings, babies sleep, nurse, and toilet. They also grow—quite quickly. The neurons in their brain connect and develop, their eyesight clarifies into full perception, and their muscles develop so that they can turn over and then crawl and then walk, run, and jump. Remarkably all this happens within the course of a year or so.

During the first year of life, children rarely place themselves into injury situations. They can't yet move into risky situations (especially in the first 6–9 months of life), and they can't yet grab dangerous objects (again, especially in the first 6–9 months of life). They also can't learn many rules or guidelines, and even if they could, adherence would be very spotty.

It is therefore largely the responsibility of parents—fatigued and emotionally drained parents—to keep their infant safe within their environments. Most infant injuries are created by caregivers. Our decisions about where we place infants and what we do with them lead to their safety or their risk for injury.

There's good news for parents, however. Infant safety is comparatively easy. You've got plenty of challenges when raising a baby from birth to her first birthday, but if you consistently follow TAMS—and during the baby years the A (act) and S (shape) components of TAMS emerge as most prominent—your baby will stay safe and grow into an injury-free toddler.

Let's discuss how you can protect your baby in various settings and locations, starting with the bedroom.

What Should I Do in the Bedroom?

Risks While Sleeping

Babies spend a lot of time sleeping, and parents get plenty of advice on how to keep babies safe while asleep. You may have heard the phrase "back to sleep," which instructs you to put your baby on his back while he sleeps. The advice is excellent because research seems to indicate that back-sleeping reduces risk of SIDS (sudden infant death syndrome).

You may also have heard that the baby's crib (and bassinet and sleeper and anywhere else the baby sleeps) should be bare. Sorry, no cute stuffed animals, blankets, bumpers, or toys—they create risk of suffocation and should be removed. If it's cold, baby sleep-sacks or warm pajamas are great choices, but even a blanket or afghan with holes is acceptable. The key is to always leave a way for your baby to breathe, reducing suffocation risks.

That also means no people in bed with the baby. Co-sleeping may be rewarding to us parents and offers great convenience for breast-feeding, but it's an unacceptable risk. There are far too many horror stories of sleeping parents rolling over and suffocating their babies to death. Don't let that happen to you. Consider a bassinet or cradle at your bedside—but no babies in your bed.

Fall Risks

Once your baby awakens, new risks arise. One of the biggest risks is falls. Consider this story from Ria:

> Wow, it's been quite a roller coaster these past four months! The first few months are a blur of feeding, diaper changing, and occasionally sleeping. Plus all the visitors: Jeremy's parents and brother and sister-in-law, his cousins, my parents, my grandma, my niece, and then all our friends. Old friends, new friends, even acquaintances who are kind-of-friends. Just a constant stream of people wanting to meet the new baby. That's great, but it was an awful lot—and I sure wasn't in the mood for entertaining. I just wanted to sleep!
>
> Then my maternity leave at work ended, and life got even more complicated. An eight-to-five job and a three-month-old girl. Really? Jeremy was a big help, and my mom was able to stay for a few weeks, but it's still a lot to manage. So I barely even registered the fact that baby Tracy was starting to roll over. I guess I kind of noticed that she would move from her back to her tummy the last few days, but it just didn't quite register for me what was happening. Jeremy said he had noticed and mentioned it to me, but that didn't hit home either. Too bad, because I really needed to know! Here's what happened.
>
> I was changing Tracy's diaper one morning. I was in a rush because I knew I would be late to work, and I was out of diapers at the changing table. There was a new box of diapers over in the closet, so I left Tracy

on the changing table and went over to the closet to resupply. I was just ripping the diaper box open and heard a loud *thump*. I turned my head and—horrors! Tracy had fallen from the changing table to the floor! I rushed over, and she was still breathing, thank God! In fact, she was crying—no surprise there—so I just held her tight. I didn't know what else to do.

After a few minutes, I called Jeremy. He had some good suggestions. First, he told me to inspect Tracy for injuries. Sure enough, there seemed to be a bump on her head. So we decided I should take Tracy to the children's hospital emergency room. I called in sick to work, got a clean diaper on Tracy (finally), and went straight to the hospital. They checked her out and told me there might be a mild concussion. Probably nothing too serious, but we needed to watch Tracy carefully for a day or two. Thankfully there were no more symptoms, and Tracy should be fine. I'm also thankful that room is carpeted—it probably softened the blow a bit.

In the end, I learned a major lesson—Tracy can roll over now, so no leaving her on the changing table unattended. I'll try to resupply the diapers better, and I'll carry her over to the closet if I ever run out of diapers again.

—Ria, mom of Tracy, age four months

Our lesson from Ria and Tracy was a good one. Once your baby gains some mobility, falls are a risk. Don't leave mobile infants unattended on changing tables, beds, sofas, or anywhere else they may fall. Anticipate potential hazards, and keep your baby secured or with you if there is any risk present.

What Should I Do in the Bathroom?

The biggest risk for infants' safety in the bathroom is at bath time. Most babies enjoy bath time. They feel warm water around them and engage closely with a loving adult. Parents also can enjoy bath time—a special moment with their young child and an opportunity to play and interact as well as clean.

Drowning risks come most often from adults who are distracted while watching children near water. A sadly all too common story runs something like this:

I was busy washing Annie's chest and tummy, and singing a little nursery rhyme to her during Sunday evening bath time. Annie was right around six months at the time. Like a lot of new moms, I was stressed and busy. I was back at work and constantly on the run. I never had any time for my husband. As I began to turn Annie over to wash her back, I heard my phone buzz on the bathroom counter. I put Annie down and looked at my phone. It was a text from my old college roommate. I hadn't heard from her in weeks, and she was telling me about her new boyfriend. I was excited to read her text and study the picture she sent. I began to type a response, and then it hit me—Annie was still in the bath!

I looked up and somehow Annie had slid down under the water. Her whole face was underwater! I panicked how could this happen? She wasn't breathing!

Luckily I somehow managed to keep my nerves. I had my phone in my hand and called 911 on speakerphone. I lifted Annie out of the water and kicked into gear—that prenatal CPR training sure was worth the time and money. The 911 operator helped, and my mouth-to-mouth resuscitation worked. Annie started breathing again. The time is all kind of a blur, but the ambulance arrived pretty quickly, and we got Annie to the hospital. The doctors say she should recover fine, hopefully without any long-term consequences at all.

What a lesson I learned. No distractions during bath time—full attention, completely and always.

—Christie, mom of Annie, age six months

Christie learned a valuable lesson, and it's one we need to share. When infants are in or near water, there must be a responsible adult supervising. That supervision must be constant and unwavering—no distractions, ever. No looking away, no walking away, and no talking away by text or voice. And one more friendly piece of advice: supervision should be sober. Save the glass of wine for after the baby goes to sleep; an intoxicated parent can make intoxicated mistakes.

There's another major risk during bath time: scald injuries. Before you put the baby in a bath, check the water temperature—each and every time, always. Hot bath water can badly hurt babies, so you must get in the habit of feeling the water, every time, before placing your baby into it.

Beyond testing the water, there's another easy trick to reduce bath-time scald risks. This is a more passive injury prevention strategy, so once you do it, you're set for a long time. Locate the water heater in your house. It's usually in your basement or a crawl space. Water heaters have a temperature dial on them. It's usually red, white, or black and looks kind of like an old-fashioned thermostat dial or gauge. Once you locate the dial, turn it down. Most experts recommend a temperature of about 120 degrees Fahrenheit (25°C), especially if there are young children in the home. Unfortunately some water heaters don't actually list temperatures, so go for somewhere closer to *warm* on the dial than *hot*. You can quickly find instructional videos online if you're not sure what to do. This passive act will greatly reduce the risk of scalds to your baby, now and throughout childhood.

Before we move from the bathroom to the kitchen, let me offer a little encouragement. Changing the temperature on your water heater is a really easy task. It literally will take you about two or three minutes but will reduce risks of scald injuries to your baby for years—and probably save you a bit of cash on the utility bills too.

What Should I Do in the Kitchen?

Eating is one of the great pleasures of life. Babies may not have language yet, but their nonverbal communication skills are often crystal clear. They seem to indicate pleasures in food and drink that match ours.

Two major risks for injury emerge surrounding the feeding of infants: scalds and choking. Let's talk about scald burns first. Whenever you feed infants—whether a newborn receiving heated formula or a nearly one-year-old chomping on microwaved chicken nuggets—you need to ensure the food isn't too hot. Follow TAMS. As your child approaches her first birthday, you can begin to teach her to touch and test food before eating it (though don't assume she will do this reliably for quite a while). You can model safe eating yourself, and you can shape behaviors of blowing, patiently waiting for food to cool (or eating cold food on the plate first), and testing food before consumption. Most important, you need to act. Consistently test food to ensure its safety before your child eats it. Yup, that means that every single time your child eats warm or hot foods, you should test the temperature first.

There is also risk of scald burns to your baby from the things you are eating and drinking yourself. We've discussed the sleep deprivation most parents of newborns face. If you're like me, you might turn to an old standby to stay alert: hot coffee or tea. The problem here won't surprise you: the mix of a tired parent, a hot cup of coffee, and a wiggly baby creates a risky concoction. The solution won't surprise you either: keep that coffee away from the baby, and perhaps keep a lid on it too. Avoid scalds by preventing them before they happen.

As your child moves into eating solid foods, the risk of choking emerges. Guidelines may make you smirk, but they are clear: grapes and hot dogs must be cut into pieces. No hard candies, popcorn, or chunks of meat and cheese. In short, cut large chunks of food into small pieces so nothing can block your child's windpipe.

What Should I Do in the Living Areas?

I apologize if this sounds patronizing, but the biggest risk to a baby in the living areas of your house is you. Parents cause injuries to their babies through negligence, ignorance, and laziness. The solutions are relatively straightforward.

Let's return to TAMS. Teaching, modeling, and shaping should be occurring, but the A for *action* is most critical here. Consider four risks.

The first risk arises while you are sitting. *Really?* You may ask. Yes. Imagine you are sitting and holding your baby. Perhaps he is drifting to sleep, perhaps he is nursing, or perhaps you are just cuddling together. It's a precious moment—you are bonding and content and happy, loving your little one. In fact, you're so content and relaxed that you yourself start to drift off to sleep. As you sleep your baby slips from your arms and crashes to the floor. Seem improbable? It happens with surprising frequency, and it can be dangerous.

Solution? If you're tired, consider your options. Could your baby sleep in the crib? Is your partner or someone else in the house who can help out while you nap? Would a caffeine or sugar jolt help?

A second risk in the living areas arises while you are walking. Again you may ask, *Really?* And again, yes. Have you ever tripped in your own house, perhaps on a loose wire, a carpet corner, or odds and ends that were left on the floor? Perhaps toys from an older sibling? In most cases you probably caught yourself before you fell to the floor, but perhaps occasionally you didn't.

Now envision those situations with a 15-pound baby in your hands. How does that change things? Even a trip where you don't fall to the floor becomes much more dangerous if you've got an infant in your arms.

Solution? Remove trip hazards from your home. Don't leave odds and ends around, and instruct older siblings to clean up their toys. Inspect for loose cords and wires, carpet corners sticking upward, and other potential hazards—then act. Remember TAMS, create a culture of safety in your household, and don't assume you'll be safe. Get those risks removed, a task that is often quick and easy.

Pay particular attention, by the way, to stairwells. Risk is multiplied on a stairway—a fall down the stairs can be fatal to an infant. Never store odds and ends on the stairway. Be sure railings are solid and stable, and use them.

The third risk is a little more personal. We all know it's dangerous to drink and drive, and we know that's because drugs and alcohol affect our judgment, reaction time, impulse control, and more. So would drugs and alcohol affect our parenting? Yes—and there's research to prove it. A single glass of wine may not significantly raise risks, but intoxicated parenting can and does have an impact on children's safety. Take care if you indulge. Funny as it may sound, choose a designated parent.

The last point I want to make extends us in a new direction. This book focuses on injuries that are unintentional. Scientists also talk about a second class of injuries: those that are intentional or the result of purposeful abuse or violence.

The line between an accidental injury and a purposeful abusive injury can be fuzzy in some cases. Consider this story from Kate:

> Another day, another blowup. My husband and I have been angry at each other for weeks, work is stressful, and money is tight. Baby Johnny was crying nonstop, and I couldn't figure out why. I tried food—no luck. I tried to rock him to sleep—no luck there either. Diaper was clean, pacifier kept getting spit out. Swaddling didn't work. I even tried that smelly stuff to

soothe gums when new teeth are coming in, and that didn't help either. I was tired, stressed, and angry at the world. No one at home to help me. Tried calling my mom—no answer. Tried my sister—no answer there either. Didn't even bother calling my husband—not worth the effort.

I can't believe I did it, but I just burst. I grabbed Johnny up and shook him and yelled at him, "Stop crying! Please!" I slapped his face a little—not too hard—and shook him in my face again. I was yelling and crying and really a bit out of control. I regret it now, but I just couldn't handle it anymore.

When my husband got home, he noticed something was wrong. I didn't really believe my husband at first, given our issues right now. But sure enough, Johnny wasn't himself—his eyes looked funny, and he didn't want to eat anything. It didn't get better the next day, so I took Johnny to the pediatrician's office. They sent me to the hospital. After a bunch of tests, the doctors said he has brain damage. I shook him too hard. I was devastated. The doctor told me Johnny might get better, but he might also have permanent damage in his brain. It could create learning problems or memory problems when he gets older. Johnny might even have hearing loss or vision loss—they need to test him for that. And they are reporting me to the state officials for suspected child abuse. A series of bad days just got worse.

—Kate, mom of Johnny, age 14 weeks

Kate was charged with child abuse, and she faced legal proceedings. Johnny's injuries were serious, affecting the rest of his life, with consequences for learning, schooling, and career. Kate was remorseful, and ethicists might debate whether her actions were intentional, but the consequences are the same. They are serious and lifelong for all involved.

The lessons from Kate are clear-cut. Babies will cry, and babies will frustrate us parents. We will get angry and stressed and upset. We will have fights with our spouses. We, the responsible adults, must nevertheless stay calm. If you feel you are about to snap, find a safe place for your child—perhaps a crib or playpen, or under the supervision of another trusted adult—and then find a way to calm yourself before resuming your parenting. We must never hurt our children.

Concluding Thoughts

Whether it's your first baby or your fifth, raising a newborn child through the first year is full of joy, happiness, and pleasure. It's also full of parenting challenges.

All four components of TAMS apply throughout childhood, but the *act* and *shape* portions of TAMS are most critical during infancy. Take action to protect your baby from the risks in her environment—from falls, choking, and scald burns. Give her a safe environment to sleep in, and remember to keep your wits to address problems calmly amid whatever fatigue, stress, and frustration you might face. Use shaping to guide your child and family to create a foundation for a culture of safety in your home. Together these steps will start your baby on a path toward safety and health throughout childhood and into adulthood.

5

TODDLER AND PRESCHOOL YEARS

Ages 1–4

B ETWEEN A CHILD'S FIRST BIRTHDAY and the start of kindergarten around age five, magic happens. A tiny baby transforms into a walking and talking being. The brain's growth is truly fantastic, and most parents find it delightful—albeit frustrating at times.

All that growth happens through extensive exploration with the world. During the toddler and preschool years, children touch, feel, taste, and explore their worlds, and that exploration can lead to injury risk. Before we talk about prevention strategies in various parts of your home and community, let's think about your child's development between the ages of one and four years old.

Cognitive Development

Cognition refers to your child's thinking abilities. The changes in cognition between age one and four are truly remarkable. Language offers an easy example. At a child's first birthday, he is just starting to learn to talk: single-word utterances might be common, but not much more. By a child's fifth birthday—wow! Children are putting together full strings of words into sentences. Four-year-olds effortlessly create sentences they have never heard before. And much to their parents' chagrin, some almost-five-year-olds might talk on and on, endlessly blabbering. Others will be quieter but still quite capable of describing their world through words.

These changes seem natural to most of us adults, but think about what has happened in your child's brain to create language. Children have learned that seemingly random mixtures of sounds form words. They have learned that words have meanings, that sounds can be merged to create words, and that words can be strung together to create sentences. They have learned the grammar of the language they speak. (Remember your lengthy verb conjugation lessons in high school foreign language classes? Your three-year-old is learning that without even trying.)

The magic of children learning language is awe inspiring, but it's far from the only cognitive skill children develop during the toddler and preschool years.

Children learn to categorize. That's relevant to safety because it helps them distinguish foods (safe and tasty to eat or drink) from poisons (dangerous to consume), which is especially important because they can't yet read labels.

Children begin to learn perspective-taking also. You and I are pretty good, for example, at figuring out when someone wants to engage with us and when they want to be left alone. Two-year-olds don't have any notion that their desires may be different from other people's desires. This ability emerges around age three or four and is mostly mastered by age five or six. How does that influence safety? Well, consider our interactions with pet dogs. You and I have a good sense of when Buddy wants to play and when he would prefer to eat or sleep. We leave Buddy alone when he's sleeping or eating, for example, and we throw a ball for him to chase when we see his tail wagging eagerly.

But if a child doesn't yet have a sense of other people's (or dogs') perspectives, she might jump on Buddy as he sleeps. That misunderstanding can lead to disaster. Consider this story from Megan:

I was lounging around watching Netflix one quiet Sunday afternoon. Lily had recently turned three, and she was playing games on her iPad in the next room. I figured she was fine to leave for a while—she loves those games and seems to play with them for hours without any problem.

All of a sudden, Spot started barking like crazy! Spot is a good dog—he hardly ever barks—and I knew something must be wrong. I rushed in to see what was going on, and I saw Lily on the floor, crying. She was bleeding too. A lot. There was blood all over the carpet, and it seemed to be coming from her forearm. Spot looked really angry and was still growling. Lily had to be my first priority, though, not Spot.

I picked Lily up and looked carefully at where the blood was coming from. I saw that Spot had bit Lily on her wrist. The bite seemed to have punctured some major arteries or veins or something, so there was lots of blood gushing out. I wrapped Lily's arm tightly with the bathroom towel to try to stop the bleeding and loaded her into the car to get her to the ER at the children's hospital. They were able to stitch her up. She'll have scars for the rest of her life, but no other long-term damage.

Once things calmed down that evening, I asked Lily what happened. She didn't remember everything, and it's hard to piece together all the details, but it seems that Lily had put down her iPad and was playing house. She had grabbed Spot's dog toy to use in her play. Spot got angry. He didn't like Lily using his toy. I guess I can understand that. Lily refused to give the toy back, and Spot bit her arm, trying to get the toy back.

> Well, there's a new rule in our house: never share toys with Spot. Spot's toys are for him, and your toys are for you. I hope Lily can remember that rule. I might have to start watching her more carefully when she plays too—I should not have left her alone in the next room while I watched Netflix.
>
> —Megan, mom of Lily, age three
> (and Spot the dog, age eight)

Megan learned some important lessons from this incident. When a child is injured, one good lesson is to seek the root of the problem. What created the injury situation? At the heart of the matter in Megan's situation was Lily's cognitive skills. At age three Lily couldn't yet understand Spot's perspective. Lily could not understand what Spot might like and dislike, and she couldn't understand that Spot wouldn't want Lily to share his toys.

What is Megan's solution? She probably needs two strategies. First, as she did, she should establish simple rules for Lily to follow, such as *no sharing toys with the dog*. Other good rules might be *no playing with Spot when he's asleep* and *no playing with Spot while he is eating*. This kind of rule-setting falls under the *s* for *shape* in our TAMS method. It helps the child learn behavior for the present and the future.

Second, Megan should act: supervise Lily more carefully when Spot is around. Even the best-trained dogs remain animals, with animal instincts. Even the smartest young children have cognitive limitations in their thinking and processing skills. Adult supervision is needed to avert tragedies.

Motor Development

Along with a growing brain, toddlers and preschoolers also have rapidly growing bodies. Parents recognize this based on their frequent trips to the shoe and clothing stores, but we injury prevention professionals also pay attention to the influence of rapid physical growth on toddlers' and preschoolers' safety.

As children grow they want to learn to use their newfound strength, size, and balance. They enjoy practicing gross motor skills, activities such as running, jumping, skipping, and hopping. Has your child ever tried to walk along the edge of a curb or a wall? That offers a great way to practice newfound and developing balancing skills. In these toddler and preschool years, children like to swing and slide and bounce and skip just about wherever they can. And in general these physical activities are healthy. They allow children to grow, develop agility, and understand the world. On occasion, however, those activities can lead to injuries.

Parents can mitigate the risk of injury by remembering TAMS. Keep an eye on your growing children, letting them explore and try new things but also "spotting" them to prevent injury as a gymnastics coach might. So let them walk along the brick wall, but keep your hand nearby to catch them in case of a slip. If they are skipping along the sidewalk, stay close to be sure they don't venture dangerously into a driveway where a car is backing out.

One caution: be judicious as a parent. You may be anxious and feel as if you need to stop your child from almost everything. Resist this temptation. Trying new physical tasks is usually healthy for your child. You should stop them when there is true risk, but let them try new things when appropriate. Follow TAMS to teach them to explore and push their bodies when the risk is acceptable, or when you can watch them enough to keep the risk acceptable. And intervene when the risk becomes too high.

Now that we understand key aspects of your child's development, let's think about ways to reduce injury risk in various parts of the house.

What Should I Do in the Kitchen?

Your exploring young child may love to play in the kitchen. Banging pots and pans, stacking plastic containers, and learning to use a spoon to eat are all great (and safe) fun! But safety risks abound in the kitchen as well. Let's discuss some simple strategies to reduce the risk.

Prevent Access

Wherever dangerous items are stored, parents should act to prevent young children's access. This means knives and other sharp kitchen instruments, cleaning supplies, dishwasher soap (yes, it's toxic even though it's used to clean), alcoholic beverages, cannabis edibles, and anything else that might harm a child.

How can you prevent access? A common strategy is through cabinet locks. These are small and low-cost plastic devices that can be installed without much difficulty. Once installed, adults know how to manipulate the levers to open the cabinet, but children usually can't figure it out. Another common strategy is to place the items up high, out of reach. This usually works too, as long as your clever child doesn't figure out how to climb on chairs and countertops to retrieve a desired item as he grows older.

Many parents assume they will always be watching and supervising, so restricting access isn't needed. This might be especially true for routine items that are used every day—it's certainly easier to just grab your daily kitchen knives from a convenient drawer without trying to negotiate cabinet locks.

Warning: this probably won't work! Many parents like you made this same mistake and regretted it after a tragedy. Even the most conscientious and careful parents will have trouble constantly supervising their young children in the kitchen. Babysitters or grandparents might be around. Parents might get distracted. Just a simple run to the doorbell or restroom can distract for a moment, and a three-year-old can open a cabinet and grab a bottle of window cleaner in seconds. Don't be sorry; take the simple steps needed to restrict access.

Preventing access taps into our TAMS method through action, but we parents can also model safety in the kitchen as our children grow through the preschool years. Use your kitchen appliances and knives safely. Most of this is common sense: cut away from your body, don't leave knives where they might fall into your feet, and use caution when removing food from the oven. Remember, your child may be watching your techniques.

And it might not hurt to teach and shape by narrating what you are doing. Here's an example: *It's time to get the cookies out of the oven. Yum, yum! Let me find a potholder to get the cookies out of the oven because they will be hot. Here it is—my favorite blue potholder. I'll put that on so I can hold the cookie tray safely, and I won't burn my hand.* Not hard, huh? Many parents might just routinely take the cookies out, but this narration is chock-full of statements that will guide and teach your little one to be a safe cook someday.

Pot Handles

Try this little experiment. Wherever you are right now, crouch down on your knees and take a look at the world the way your child sees it. Things look different, don't they? You're now looking up at things that you used to look down upon. And you've lost perspective to see other things.

OK, good. Now try doing this same experiment in front of your stovetop. Spin the handle of a pot or pan outward, hanging over the edge. Your short-heighted children can see this handle, can't they? But they don't know what is in the pot or pan. They just see a black or silver handle protruding outward. And we all know young children are curious—they want to understand and explore their world. So guess what. Yup. Grab the handle and pull.

If the pot is empty, we might just have a loud noise, or we might have a pot land on our head, creating a concussion risk. If the pot or pan is filled with boiling spaghetti or hot soup, we've got a serious risk of scald burns.

What's the solution? Another easy one. Adopt the habit of turning your pot and pan handles inward. Every time. That way they're out of view of your curious toddlers and preschoolers. They're out of reach also. This is really an easy one, folks—just get in the habit of pointing those handles inward to avert injuries.

Hot Liquids

We talked about the risks of hot foods to infants in the last chapter. Don't stop paying attention to scald-burn risks when your child celebrates her first birthday. The same two risks persist: burns from your own food or drink and burns from food or drink for your child.

If you're like me, those sleepless nights caring for an infant may have increased (or kickstarted) your coffee habit. To paraphrase the coffee ads, for many of us a steaming-hot cup of coffee is the best way to wake up and start the day. We just need to make sure the hot coffee doesn't end up on our child, where it could scald the skin.

As your child grows older, the secret is to be aware. Always. Whenever you have hot coffee—or tea or soup or anything else—think about where it is, and think about where your child is. Remember the old adage "Expect the unexpected," and act to promote safety. If your coffee is on the coffee table, your curious child might grab it and spill it on herself. Move it higher. If your hot soup sits on the kitchen table and your child is hungry, it might land on him. Always remember that children in this age group will grab, explore, and taste. So keep the hot liquids separate from the curious children, and injuries will be avoided.

Keeping your children safe from burning themselves with their own food is simple too. Let's hear from Sunita on this one.

I love my son, Rohit, so much, but I have to admit he is a bit of a grumpy waker-upper. I think he got that from my husband. First thing in the morning, he will come down to our bed and whine and moan for no particular reason. The best way to stop it is to give him food—once he's got something in his stomach, he becomes our cute and loving boy again.

So I've started giving him oatmeal in the morning. It's quick and easy: pour the mix into a bowl, add some milk, nuke it in the microwave for 30 seconds, and it's set to go. Sometimes I even get fancy and sprinkle some cinnamon on top for him.

This morning we started with the usual pattern. Rohit came down to our bed and started whining, and I robotically went into the kitchen to prepare the oatmeal. Mix cereal and milk in the bowl, push the buttons to start the oatmeal, add a spoon, and throw it all on the table for him. Then start making my coffee and breakfast.

Rohit took the first bite and shrieked. I rushed over and he yelled, "Hot!" I put my lips to the oatmeal on his spoon and sure enough, it was hot—way too hot even for me. Not sure what happened—maybe my hand slipped and I microwaved the oatmeal for 60 seconds instead of 30? The six is right below the three on the number pad. I'm not sure.

Rohit was OK, but I learned a lesson. I'll always check the temperature before I give him his food. And I'll watch the numbers on the microwave as I punch them in.

—Sunita, mom of Rohit, age two

We can all benefit from Sunita's lessons, and most parents have learned similar ones. Always test your child's hot food before she eats it to avoid minor and major burn injuries. For that matter, test your own food also. It's a great way to model and shape safety as you create the culture of safety you desire in your home.

What Should I Do in the Bathroom?

The risks to your toddler or preschooler in the bathroom are actually somewhat similar to those in the kitchen. Think about where and how things are stored. Anything dangerous—and there's usually plenty of that in a bathroom—needs to be inaccessible. In fact, you're probably even less likely to be supervising your child carefully in a bathroom than you are in a kitchen, so be sure to check and double-check that your dangerous items are stored safely. What goes on the list? Obviously the cleaning supplies. But think also about soaps and shampoos, makeup, medications (over-the-counter and prescription), and scissors, tweezers, and razors. Most of those things can be risky to children. Some can be fatal. Your options? Follow TAMS and act the same as you did in the kitchen: install cabinet locks or move things to high shelves.

Another risk in the bathroom is drowning. When we picture the tragedy of a child drowning, we often imagine beaches or swimming pools. But a surprising number of young children drown in the home, regrettably in small amounts of water and in mundane places such as buckets and pails, toilet bowls, and bathtubs. The prevention strategies here are also easy actions: empty your buckets and pails, close your toilet lids, and drain your bathtubs.

Of course, supervision is also critical. But recognize the challenges of constant supervision, as we've discussed, and take the simple steps to reduce risk by removing dangerous water sources from your children's home environment.

What Should I Do in the Playroom? My Child's Bedroom?

Play is intertwined with childhood. Every child in every culture plays. Play helps children learn. It helps children explore. And it helps children grow.

So how can we, as parents, encourage safe and healthy play in our children? Let's think about a few aspects of children's play and how we can teach, act, model, and shape to make the setting—whether it be a playroom, a child's bedroom, or any other indoor setting—safe for play.

Toys

The first step is to make sure the child's toys are safe. We hear about risks periodically in the popular media: choking hazards from small parts, swallowed batteries and magnets, lead paint, and so on. We also hear about toy recalls. How's a parent to keep it all straight?

Lucky for us, a lot of risks are handled through the age recommendations that appear on toy boxes. Don't ignore those labels. If a toy says it is for ages six and up, don't give it to your four-year-old. If you buy or inherit used toys, take care and figure out what age the toy is intended for. There's a reason for the age suggestions, and most often it is to protect children's safety.

Batteries are truly dangerous for young children. Swallowed batteries can be fatal. That's why newer toys have difficult-to-change battery compartments. A generation or two ago, kids just popped batteries in and out of their toys themselves. But as doctors and scientists have recognized the risks of batteries—especially small coin-cell batteries—we now recommend that adults always help young children with battery changes. This offers a great opportunity to model and shape how we handle potentially dangerous objects carefully, so try to involve your children in battery changes for their toys. When they are young, have them watch you model safe behavior. As they grow older, shape their behavior by allowing them to help, eventually allowing them to make the battery change while you supervise. This is the art of shaping to create a culture of safety: teach, model, and supervise while the child tries.

Toy recalls are frustrating to parents and children alike. Who wants to return or repair a beloved toy? Also frustrating is sorting out which particular toys are recalled. There are lists available on various websites, including the US Consumer Product Safety Commission, but who has the time to hunt those lists down and then compare the long lists to the inventory of toys present in the household? One easy recommendation is to complete the product registration information that comes in the packaging. If you've registered a new product and it gets recalled, the manufacturer will let you know.

Once you are aware a toy has been recalled, you need to take action. This step may or may not be complicated. If returning the item is required to obtain a replacement, your child may not want to give it up. If repairs are required, you may be sent some parts and then have to complete the repair yourself. In the end we return to the *A* in TAMS: act to follow through with toy recalls. Act also by safeguarding and supervising. Keep an eye on your children while they play.

The Room

OK, so you've got safe toys in the room. You'll do your best to supervise your child while he plays. Is there anything you should do to playrooms and children's bedrooms to make them safer?

Yes. Among the easiest-to-install and cheapest-to-purchase child safeguarding devices are outlet covers. You probably know what they are: small plastic doohickeys that you plug into an outlet so that a child can't put her finger, toy, screwdriver, or anything else into it. Simple, easy, and affordable—get them purchased and installed.

And don't forget to reinstall, either. Consider this story from Jerome:

Saturday. Cleaning day in our household. My wife was downstairs working on laundry and dishes, and keeping an eye on three-year-old Saul. Baby Samuel, just two months old, was napping.

My job was vacuuming. I don't mind that task—gives me a little bit of exercise (and yes, I sure need that!), and it kind of feels good to finish one room and move to the next. I was downstairs working on the basement playroom. That's the hardest room in the house to vacuum probably—have to pick up all the toys that are thrown all over to even reach the carpet and get it vacuumed. I got the floor cleared, took the outlet cover off, and plugged the vacuum in. *Vrmmm*—it was whirring away. I got the room all vacuumed and turned it off. Then I heard my wife yelling—apparently baby Samuel had woken up, and she had her hands full. I pulled up the cords of the vacuum, put it away, and zipped upstairs. Did not even think about the outlet cover!

A few days later, I got home from work, and my wife gave me a stern look and pulled me aside, away from the kids. She was definitely not in the usual loving mood I expect when I get home from work. She explained how she had gone down to get Saul for a snack, and he had his plastic toy adventure character in his hand. The toy was reaching into the outlet socket, and Saul was playing as if the toy doll was getting power for his next superhero mission. Oh no! I couldn't believe it. I accidentally left the outlet uncovered, and Saul saw it and started playing with it right away.

We were lucky the toy was plastic; the electricity didn't conduct through it. Saul wasn't hurt at all. But I sure learned an important lesson. Outlet covers are there for a reason, and they need to be reinstalled without error.

—Jerome, dad of Saul, age three, and Samuel, two months

What Should I Do on the Stairway?

As children learn to walk, they often stumble and fall. This is fine and normal in most household settings, but not on a stairway. Falls down stairways can be very serious and even fatal, so parents must take steps to prevent their young children from falling down stairs.

There's one important message to start with: falls can happen as your child goes down *or* up the stairs. And the falls can be equally dangerous. If you fall down eight stairs, it doesn't matter much if you were on your way down them or on your way up; either fall can be quite dangerous.

So what should parents do? Act. The best strategy is to block access. Install a stair gate that keeps children on the same level of the home. Stair gates are a little convoluted to install sometimes but well worth the effort. Act also to remove odds and ends from the stairway. Keep the path clear so no one trips.

And remember all your other TAMS strategies too. Model safety by using the handrails when you go up and down stairs yourself. Even if you don't need them, your child will benefit as she grows. To shape, enforce your household rules and lessons about holding hands with an adult while going up and down stairs, clearing junk off the stairway, and using handrails. Ultimately your behavior on the stairs will merge with your behavior throughout the house to create your household's culture of safety.

What Should I Do in the Yard?

How can you learn about the world if you don't explore the world? As children explore their world, they venture to new places, try new things, and push their physical limits. In a lot of cases, this is perfectly fine. But when the exploration is in your yard, risks emerge. Consider this story from Jennifer, which is far too common:

I'll never forget that terrible fall weekend. My husband and I were in the den, watching a football game and having a few drinks. Another couple was at our place with us. They live just down the street, and we often hang out together on the weekends. Our older boy was in his room playing video games with the other couple's son.

Jeff was in his room playing Legos—or at least we thought he was. He loved Legos, and we never had any worries at all when he played with them because he could do it forever. He would build trucks and buildings and roads—really he would build whole cities and just play with them for hours. But for some reason that afternoon, it seems he wandered off into the yard. I don't know why. I wish I could ask him. I wish I had told him to play Legos in the den with us. Or play video games with the older boys. But we didn't do that.

The football game ended. Our team won, and I called the boys down for a snack. The two older ones rushed in to eat. They were hungry. Jeff didn't come, so I called again. Still no response. After a third try, I walked upstairs to get him. He wasn't in his room. I asked the older boys where he was, and they didn't know. Everyone started searching the house—no luck. My husband had the first thought to try outside, and that's when our concern turned to tragedy.

Jeff was at the bottom of the swimming pool. My husband jumped in, clothes and all, to rescue him. But it was too late. CPR didn't help. The paramedics arrived and tried to revive him. It didn't work. Jeff was gone at the precious age of three years, four months, and eight days old. He'll never come back.

It still doesn't seem possible. I cry every day. All we have left is our memories. And his Legos. I will always and forever keep the last Lego truck he made that afternoon. It's right next to my bed—the last thing I look at when I go to sleep, and the first thing I look at when I wake up.

What happened? I don't exactly know. Jeff somehow wandered outside. The gate to the pool area was left open, and he just walked right in. No one knows why he went there or what he was doing or how he ended up in the pool. All his clothes were still on, so I guess he somehow slipped. I don't think he wanted to go swimming. He didn't really know how to swim, and he couldn't reach the bottom, so once he was in the water, I'm sure everything happened real quick.

—Jennifer, mom of Jeff, deceased at age three,

and Paul, age eight

Of course, swimming pools aren't the only dangers. Lakes, rivers, creeks, and streams also present risk outside, in and near some yards. And other risks can also emerge: falls from trees, wild animal bites, and more.

The TAMS method can guide us in three areas for prevention.

First, supervise. Young children do not have the thinking skills to keep themselves safe. They are impulsive, have poor judgment, and do not think about the consequences of their decisions. This isn't really their fault—it's just the way children's brains work until they get older. So adults must make decisions for children. We need to oversee how they act and what they do, and we must rescue children from poor decisions and actions. When it comes to engaging near water, the risks involved are significant, so supervision needs are amplified. Children just cannot be left alone when drowning risks are present. Supervision must be constant, attentive, and intense.

Second, safeguard. In Jeff's case someone made a tragic mistake by leaving the pool gate open. Many jurisdictions now mandate fencing around backyard swimming pools, but such fencing is useless if gates are left ajar. More generally, safeguarding can take many forms: locked doors, closed gates, door alarms, and other means to prevent access to water and other risks are obvious. Other strategies might be subtler: ropes dividing shallow and deep swimming areas reduce risk among older toddlers and preschoolers, for example.

Third, teach. Toddlers are capable of learning and following a small number of basic rules, so teach them what they need to know: swim only when an adult is present, and don't enter a swimming area without an adult. Other yard-safety guidelines might include how high up a tree a child can safely climb and how to react when locally present dangerous wild animals, snakes, or insects appear.

It's also important to teach your child to swim. Some experts argue that swimming lessons should be universally required; scientific research suggests knowing how to swim does reduce drowning risks. Plus there's a happy bonus: children enjoy swimming!

What Should I Do in the Neighborhood?

Streets and Traffic

Most adults cross streets without a lot of thought, but crossing a street is a complex task that strains children's limited capacity. In fact, most experts agree that toddlers and preschoolers simply do not have the cognitive skills to engage safely in traffic. And they are too young to learn those skills. This means parents must implement the TAMS method to help children when they walk, bike, skate, skateboard, or otherwise engage in and near traffic.

Let's review the full TAMS method and how it might apply to traffic situations. First, we teach. Teach children to look for traffic, and teach them to think about the speeds and distances of oncoming vehicles. Teach them also how traffic signals work: what red and green lights mean, and what "walk" and "don't walk" signals look like. But as you teach, remember that young children will only absorb and remember bits and pieces of what you tell them. Early lessons are extremely valuable, but children are unlikely to safely engage independently in traffic until at least age eight or nine, and often later than that.

Because teaching will not create safety, let's think about the *A* in TAMS: *act*. We must safeguard the environment: supervise children to stay in safe areas when they walk (on sidewalks, no crossing streets alone) and bike (in parks or away from traffic, and always wearing protective equipment such as helmets).

How about *M*, for *model*? Absolutely we can and should model safety near traffic. It's easy for parents to slip up on this one too. Don't jaywalk—your children will notice. Don't walk across streets while distracted by your phone—children will notice this also! Wear a helmet if you bicycle, and follow traffic laws when you bike and drive. Don't underestimate the power of modeling around traffic. Your children are watching you.

Finally, let's think about *shaping*. Here we return to our long-term effort to guide, coax, and monitor our children for safe behavior, working to create a culture of safety in our household. How do we do this? Set rules about safe engagement in and near traffic, and enforce them. Hold hands in parking lots (they're surprisingly dangerous at this age). Look both ways together (yes, that means you remind your child to look both ways) before crossing any streets. Reward obedience—again, that's most important to shape a culture of safety—and gently reprimand nonadherence. Be consistent too. Never ever permit exceptions, such as bicycling helmetless, even for short trips or in "safe" places.

If you can follow TAMS, you will help your toddler grow into a safe preschooler and then a safe school-aged child. This will lead naturally into—scary as it may seem, it will come sooner than you realize—a safe teen driver and an adult who practices safety in daily life. You'll be on the path to a culture of safety in your household.

Playground

There's one other neighborhood destination that we should discuss: playgrounds. Today's playgrounds are increasingly safe—mostly gone are the days of concrete pads under the swing sets, hot metal sliding boards, and jungle gyms that reach the sky. But that doesn't mean playgrounds are without risks.

The first thing parents should do is recognize what is age appropriate for their children. Many of today's larger playgrounds are built with two or more sections, each for a different age group. There may be one section for younger children and one for older children. Learn which is which. And here's the hard part: teach your child to play only on the section that fits her age group.

Then parents should supervise. There are a few ways to supervise. One is to actually engage and play with your child on the playground. Remember, the physical activity is good for you too. The other is to let your child run and play—that's healthy too—and for you to keep an eye on things so you can intervene if a risky situation is impending. Proper supervision means no phones, though. Full attention and preparedness to intervene will be necessary if one child is darting in front of another on the swing set, preparing to jump from an eight-foot height, or throwing sand or mulch toward another.

When risks occur, enter your shaping mode—promptly intervene, explain the risks, and redirect your child to a safer activity. Don't go overboard—playground time should be fun and disciplining minimized. For comparatively minor infractions, which describes most playground events, simply stay calm, redirect, and let your child keep playing. Remember that rewarding positive and safe play is the best route to household safety. Punishing negative behaviors is always less effective.

Concluding Thoughts

The toddler and preschool ages are joyous for children and their parents. Reflect upon the joys you are experiencing: learning colors, numbers, and letters; exploring and understanding our majestic world, with all its beautiful sights, sounds, smells, and tastes; learning to move, jump, climb, and discover; developing friendships, relationships, and love for one's family.

All that exploration does create risk, especially in our modern and complex world. The TAMS method will help create a culture of household safety during these years. Teach your children basic rules. Act to safeguard the environment and supervise your children near risks. Model safe behavior. And slowly, patiently, and calmly shape your children into who you want them to be—children who explore, discover, and experiment in the world, but who do so safely, as they grow.

6

THE EARLY
SCHOOL YEARS

Ages 5–8

DO YOU REMEMBER your first day of kindergarten? The question may conjure nostalgic thoughts. The start of school and formal learning. New friends, new places, and new experiences. Songs, sights, and learning to read. The list might go on, but one message is clear: the start of formal schooling marks a major transition in our lives.

Along with the start of schooling come major changes in how children think and how they engage with peers and adults. Let's consider some of those changes and how they might influence child safety and injury prevention.

Perception and Judgment

Early in my career, while I was still a PhD student, I conducted an experiment with guidance from my dissertation advisor, Dr. Jodie Plumert. The experiment was fairly simple. We asked children to complete four basic physical tasks. For example, they had to stand behind one wooden stick and step over a second parallel wooden stick without jumping. In another task children stood on their tiptoes and reached up to retrieve a cute little rubber frog off a high shelf. Sometimes the tasks were set up to be within the child's ability to complete, and sometimes they were beyond the child's physical abilities.

Before children tried each task, we asked them to look at the task and judge whether they could complete it. Guess what? Kids overestimated what they could do. They felt they could step and reach much farther than they actually could. In fact, even adults overestimated their own abilities to some extent, but children overestimated much more frequently. And the younger the children, the more they overestimated their abilities.

Another really interesting result also emerged. The children who overestimated the most had a history of getting hurt the most. That's right: overestimation of ability to complete tasks—misperceiving one's ability—was related to injury history.

Now, you might be thinking: these results are not much of a surprise. Of course children think they can do more than they can. That's the only way they can learn about the world. We need to push ourselves to learn and grow. The only way we learn to walk is by taking the first step. The only way we learn to shoot a basketball is by taking that first shot. The only way we learn to drive is by turning the key in the ignition for the first time. All correct and all true. Child development is indeed about developing, and we need to try things to grow. As our experiment showed, humans do have a natural inclination to perceive they can do things that might be out of reach.

There's an important caveat, however. When we misperceive something that could cause injury, we make too much of a leap. We need to try things with some degree of caution and with some ability to temper and restrain ourselves when an action might lead to injury.

Dr. Plumert, my students, and I conducted several more of those types of experiments, trying to find good ways to discourage children from taking risks. We tried asking the children to stop and think about their decision for a few seconds before acting. That didn't help much. We tried having the children watch other children take risks. That didn't help either—in fact, children tended to copy the others and take the same risks.

We did reduce overestimation of ability through one strategy: putting parents in the room. When children knew their parents (usually Mom) were watching, they took fewer risks. This was true even when the parents didn't communicate with the children—the parents just stood quietly in the back of the room, where no verbal or visual communication could occur. And remarkably the most impulsive and risk-taking children were the ones who were most influenced by the presence of their parents. So the most injury-prone children were the ones whose risk-taking reduced the most when a parent was watching.

There's a critical message for all of us parents here: children notice our presence, and they are more cautious when they know we are watching them. When we act by supervising, children take note.

Social Development

A quick review of what we just learned:

1.   Children overestimate their ability to complete basic physical tasks such as stepping and reaching. They think they can step and reach farther than they actually can. This is healthy because it allows growth and development, but it also can lead to unfortunate injuries when children overestimate their ability to complete tasks that are dangerous.
2.   Adult supervision offers a simple and effective strategy to reduce children's overestimation of ability. When children know they are

being watched, they take fewer risks. And the children who are most influenced by this are the same children who tend to take the most risks—the most impulsive and risk-taking children.

Interestingly our research has shown this behavior pattern not just in a laboratory but also near traffic, with parents watching children cross pretend streets. When children knew their parents were watching carefully, they displayed safer pedestrian behavior. And we extended the pattern beyond parents. It seemed to influence preschoolers when their teachers started watching the playground more carefully. It influenced 9- and 10-year-old youth soccer players too: with more referees on the field watching them, they committed fewer aggressive fouls. And it influenced children of all ages at a public swimming pool: when the lifeguards started watching more carefully, the children took fewer risks while they were swimming.

These results prove that children are influenced by the people near them. If parents or other adults watch children carefully, the adults can prevent children from doing something dangerous. Adults have the clear advantages of more-developed abilities to think (cognition) and judge (perception) and therefore can better sense when something might be safe versus when it might lead to injury. But supervision has effects that go beyond simple intervention to stop a child from doing something dangerous. Supervision also seems to cause children to take fewer risks. When children know they are being watched, they engage in their world more safely.

Of course, social influences on children's behavior are not limited to the influences of parents. Schoolchildren spend plenty of time with peers outside the supervision of adults, and in those instances peer influences may have particularly powerful effects on behavior. Consider Sid's story:

I'm just about done with second grade. I'm lucky because a bunch of my friends from school live right in my neighborhood. We hang out together all the time. Joe, Ken, and Lou are my closest buddies.

Right now it's late spring. Where I live, it rains a lot in spring, so the creek in our neighborhood is running real quick. On weekends in spring, Joe, Ken, Lou, and I love to play near the creek. We search for frogs and chase squirrels and build forts. Sometimes we play tag or other games.

Last weekend we were playing tag. I was "it," so I was chasing after the others. They're all second-graders too, but they are a little taller than me. My mom says it's my genetics. I've always been the short kid in the class. Anyway Joe, Ken, and Lou were running away from me because I was it, and they came up to the creek. When the water is low, it's easy to cross the creek just about anywhere. But it's spring, so the water was high and there were fewer choices. You can go down to the log bridge, but that's pretty far away. You can go to the bridge where the road is, but that's really far away too, in the other direction. Another choice is to try to jump across the whole creek at its narrowest point, but even Lou has trouble doing that—and he's the tallest and most athletic of all of us. The high schoolers do that, but not us. The last choice is to jump the rocks. There are three rocks that kind of make a path across the water, but they are slippery and far apart.

Well, I was chasing after Joe, Ken, and Lou, and they got to the creek and started running toward the rocks. I was going after them. Lou was first. When he got to the rocks, he hopped right across like always. He always makes it look so easy. Then Joe and Ken tried it. They went a little slower, but they made it too. I was scared. I've never tried the rocks. But I didn't want to stay behind, and if I went down to one of the bridges, I'd have no hope to get across and tag someone. Plus the other kids were on the other side of the creek, kind of making fun of me and kind of egging me on. I had to try it.

I took it slow. I jumped to the first rock safely. Then I went to go to the second one, and I slipped. It was too far! I fell right into the creek. It was cold, and my pants and shoes were all dirty and wet. I could reach the bottom, so I just kind of limped out of the water. My friends were laughing at me. Laughing hard! My ankle hurt because of the way I hit the rock before I slipped. I looked silly, and I was shivering. I quit the game and headed home to get cleaned up and tell my mom what happened.

I guess I was lucky. I didn't get hurt bad. I should've known I was too short to jump the rocks. But I wanted to prove to my friends that I could jump the rocks like they did.

—Sid, age seven

Sid's situation is not unusual—peers are likely to encourage other peers to take risks. Sid wasn't hurt bad, but sometimes the consequences can be much more serious. And this horrifies us parents. What can we as parents do to keep our children safe when we are not there to protect them? As children grow older, this situation becomes increasingly common. The answer lies in our TAMS method, and especially in the teaching, modeling, and shaping we have done.

To keep our children safe when they are not with us, we need them to make the right decisions on their own, without us. Fortunately we shape them to do that. We teach them safety, we model safe behaviors, and we shape their behavior into our household culture of safety. Sid may actually have recognized there was some chance he would fall into the creek, but he also knew that would just get him muddy and wet, not put him at risk for a serious injury. In a different circumstance, where serious injury was possible, Sid may possibly have made the safer decision.

Shaping children to be safe is tough work. It happens over the course of weeks and months and years, and it requires patience and persistence. Remember also that it's never too late to start shaping. Shaping is truly a process that happens constantly, throughout your children's development. If your child is like Sid—perhaps a bit smaller or a bit clumsier than his friends—you can discuss with him that peers may have expectations he can't meet. Give your child the confidence to say no and to find good alternatives to thorny situations like the one Sid faced.

No matter what your child is like, work with her to recognize peer influences. Role-play possible scenarios, and practice restraint, friendly rejection, and seeking of alternatives. Set rules and enforce them consistently. Set expectations and reward children for meeting them.

TAMS for Early School-Age Children

The TAMS method crosses all age groups, but the early school years represent a time when it really kicks in for both children and parents. It's truly an exciting time in a child's life.

Teaching becomes somewhat easier for parents because children learn to learn, and learn to listen to teachers, in a formal elementary school setting. They develop more patience to absorb lessons and then to try out those lessons in the real world. They still make plenty of mistakes, though—rules are forgotten and disregarded—so parents should be patient (repeated lessons are needed) and observant (close supervision is still needed in risky settings).

A parent's actions will transition during children's early school years too. Some of the home safety devices you installed can be dismantled; most parents eagerly celebrate the removal of stair gates, for example, as stairway fall risks decrease sharply. Another welcome change at this age is the graduation out of car seats into booster seats. Broadly, supervision duties may ease a touch but only slowly and cautiously, as the safety-related decision-making of early elementary school students remains questionable.

The modeling portion of TAMS never really goes away, all the way through your child's adolescence and young adulthood. Indeed, it doesn't even change much. If you behave safely, your child will learn to behave safely. If you create a culture of safety in your home, your child will absorb it. That goes for a two-year-old, a seven-year-old, or a fifteen-year-old. So stay safe yourself. Modeling is easy. It doesn't require any language, teaching, or instructions of any type. Your child will simply observe and learn from what you do.

Shaping also continues throughout a child's development, but the early elementary school years offer a golden opportunity for parents to shape their children's behavior for the future. This is a great time for parents to set a reasonable number of safety-related rules and truly enforce them, calmly and consistently. Remember to praise and reward safe behaviors—quick verbal messages and little hugs and kisses will do the trick—as a first priority. Use firm or angry discipline much more sparingly and only when needed.

Enjoy these glory years of childhood, when youthful innocence remains prominent but learning and growing happen quickly. Instill a culture of safety in your house; those lessons will remain with your child for a lifetime and, stating it extremely but truthfully, you may even save your child's life.

Let's talk now about some specific actions you can take in various parts of your home, yard, and neighborhood.

What Should I Do in the Kitchen?

Evolution placed food among humans' greatest satisfactions, along with sex, water, and shelter. We can't subsist long without eating. It's not surprising, therefore, that many children become intrigued with cooking.

We should encourage children to learn the pleasures of a kitchen, but we must do so with attention to the risks involved. Sharp blades (think: knives) and heat (think: ovens and stovetops) are most concerning. TAMS helps.

Of course, we must model safe behavior in the kitchen. We must also begin to teach. Safe use of knives is actually rather simple to teach because dull knives can cut soft foods without significant risk (consider starting with a butter knife cutting butter, then moving to a dulled knife cutting soft cheese, proceeding step-by-step to a sharp knife cutting vegetables or meats). Increasingly sharp knives may be used only after children demonstrate mastery of the duller ones.

Safe negotiation of hot ovens and stovetops is a little trickier to teach. Lots of modeling will help—what to do in each instance and how to cope with surprises and emergencies (heavy pans, splashing grease, and so on). This is another case where you might actually explicitly teach while modeling. Talk out what you are doing to be safe as you negotiate hot foods and appliances. Over time lessons can progress to closely supervised action. Let your child practice with cold items (as a start, remove room-temperature bread from a room-temperature toaster oven, for example, before graduating to toast that has been toasted).

Shaping may be the most critical step in the kitchen. What are the rules and guidelines about how, where, and when to use knives? Which potholders should be worn, always, to reach into an oven? How should pot handles be arranged on a stovetop? (Hint: always inward.) Teach, remind, and enforce kitchen rules to instill a safety mindset.

And who knows? With time and luck, in another few years you may be the proud recipient of a birthday breakfast in bed, hand-prepared in your kitchen by your preteen child!

What Should I Do in the Bathroom?

Some good news: injury risks in the bathroom decrease as your child grows older. Supervision may still make sense in the bathtub during the early elementary school years, especially if your child doesn't yet know how to swim, but that can decrease as your child develops, and certainly if your child transitions from baths to showers.

Cabinet locks in the bathroom (and other locations) where dangerous household items are present may still make sense, but these can also be removed as your child grows older, gains the ability (and knowledge) to read labels, and becomes sophisticated enough to accurately judge what is safe and not safe to eat or drink.

What Should I Do on the Stairway?

More good news here: stairway fall risk is decreasing, and you should be able to remove stair gates. Keep striving to leave your stairways clear of the junk that always seems to accumulate (at least in my household), and continue shaping key rules about traveling up and down stairs: no jumping, no running, no playing.

What Should I Do in the Playroom?

As your child grows older, unsupervised play will be more common. For this reason, safeguarding—in the playroom and actually the whole house—remains important. Firearms and medications should be locked up. Toys in the playroom should be toys for children in the right age group. Rules should be created for how and when to play as well as who is involved in what play activities.

In fact, rules, the basis for shaping your child's behavior, should constitute a major strategy for safety promotion surrounding play in the early school years. Without harping, annoying, or harshly disciplining, children should be frequently, gently, and lovingly reminded of where and how they can play, and where and how they cannot. Intermittent supervision should occur, and children should be praised when they are playing well, according to the rules. Friendly suggestions of activities and periodic engagement of parents with their children is healthy: encourage and direct children's play to activities you feel are healthful and away from those that might be less so.

As an example, you might frequently discover during solo playtime that your child turns to video games or iPads for entertainment. This is fine—children can learn valuable skills from technology—but you'll probably agree with me that too much screen time is bad for any child. So suppose you walk in to check on your child in the playroom and discover she is watching amateur music videos on her iPad that might promote risk-taking. Which of these responses might be more effective?

> *Too much screen time! Get off your iPad and find something else to do!*

> *Wow, you've been on your iPad for a while, haven't you? What do you say we play a board game together? I like these two. Which one would you rather play?*

The second option, of course, is likely to be more effective in yielding a change in behavior, moving the child to a healthier activity. Unfortunately reality is such that our parent lives are hectic, and lying on the floor to play a quiet board game after dinner just doesn't fit into the schedule all the time. So we might try this alternative response instead:

> *Wow, you've been on your iPad for a while, haven't you? Let's look in the cabinet and see what else you might do. Hmm . . . here's an arts and crafts kit. Or a jigsaw puzzle. Or this looks interesting—some science experiments for kids. Which of those three do you want to try? The arts and crafts, the puzzle, or the science experiments?*

Why might that work? First, it redirects the child away from the iPad and to an alternative, healthier activity. Second, it offers the child control of the situation—it lets her decide which activity to engage in. The parent would be happy with any of the three options, all of which remove the child from the risk-taking iPad videos. But by giving the child control to make a decision, the parent pushes her into a healthy activity that she selected rather than one her parent imposed on her. Third, it allows the parent to get his own tasks accomplished with minimal supervision of the child.

A few caveats. First, this means you have activities such as arts and crafts, jigsaw puzzles, and science experiments available in your household. Remember that detail during the next holiday or birthday season. Second, it presumes your child has been shaped to respond to your suggestions and will engage in one of the alternative activities. Be persistent, and over time your child will become accustomed to such suggestions and react positively. Allowing some screen time—mixed judiciously with alternatives—is also likely to yield greater success than complete prohibition of what your child might prefer (and what your child talks to peers at school about).

What Should I Do in the Yard?

The great outdoors, including our own yards and neighborhood parks, are full of all sorts of hazards: trees to climb, snakes that bite, and roadways to explore. Active supervision is your best strategy when children play outdoors, but depending on your type of yard and community, it may be safe to allow children in the early elementary years to play unsupervised at times. Having fences to keep them close is a big help. Establishing a culture of safety through TAMS, with strongly shaped behavior to follow established rules, also helps. Of course, your modeling of safe play outdoors provides valuable lessons as well.

One major risk to children in this age group is the risk of drowning. Whether you have a backyard pool or not, if your child hasn't yet learned to swim by the time he enters first grade, it's time. Knowing how to swim can save a life.

However, knowing how to swim does not address all risks. Consider this story from Eduardo, the father of three:

Summer is my favorite season of the year. Work duties are lighter, and the kids are off school. We spend just about every summer weekend down at the lake. I love taking the kids fishing and swimming, and the whole family enjoys the relaxing atmosphere on the water.

The kids are like dolphins—they've been excellent swimmers since they were really young. But we always put safety first anyway. Life jackets are required when you ride on the boat. And no kids swim without an adult watching.

One hot August afternoon, I took the kids out on the boat. My wife decided to stay back at the lake house and read a book on the deck. Nothing was too unusual. We were cruising around, and everyone was wearing their life jackets, enjoying the scenery and laughing. We decided to drop anchor and jump in the lake to cool off.

And that was the mistake. When we swim in the lake, we usually take our life jackets off—it's easier to move around and play in the water without them on, and everyone is a strong swimmer and watching out for each other.

But this stupid Jet Skier came speeding by. Boy, was he stupid. He was driving recklessly and superfast, and not paying attention. He came straight toward Eddy—he was within inches of running him over. Literally just inches! Luckily Eddy saw the Jet Ski coming and dove underwater as far as he could. He wasn't hit by the Jet Ski. I think it went right over the top of him. Smart kid. And quick thinking. When he popped back up, I was so relieved. I've never felt like that in my life. I thought Eddy might be gone forever. Whew.

> We've learned some lessons. First, only swim in designated areas, where the water is roped off from stupid boaters and Jet Skiers. Second, always wear life jackets on the water. It is just too risky to take them off, even when you are a strong swimmer. Third, pay attention. This whole thing wasn't my fault or Eddy's fault either. The Jet Skier was reckless and stupid. But Eddy was paying attention, and it may have saved his life.
>
> —Eduardo, dad of Julia, age nine,
> Eddy, age six, and Juan, age four

As Eduardo's story illustrates, drowning risk among school-age children occurs in a variety of circumstances and environments. Children can be alone, with peers, or supervised by adults. They can be in backyard swimming pools, at beaches, on lakes, or in any number of other settings. Kids living on farms have even been known, sadly, to drown in manure pits.

So what's a parent to do? Follow TAMS.

Teach. Teach your children to swim, and teach them rules for water safety. Teach them to think about their world and the consequences that might result from risky actions. As Eduardo learned, teach your children to swim only in safe places. Swimming in a marked swim area would have protected Eddy and his family.

Act. Eduardo recognized the importance of supervision. Adults need to watch children while they are in and near water. Foresee potential risks and take action to stop dangerous activities. Also, avoid distractions while you supervise. An adult scrolling on his phone is useless if a child is drowning. Act also to safeguard. When the kids are finished in the backyard kiddie pool, dump the water out to avoid a tragedy. Put fencing around backyard pools, and cover hot tubs. Foresee potential risks, and take action to prevent accidents before they happen.

Model. From a very young age, children learn by watching the behavior of those they trust and respect. If parents don't wear life jackets on the boat, children likely won't either. If parents swim past the buoys at the beach, their children may do so also. If parents flaunt rule-breaking, their children will as well. So, hard as it may be, you must always remember that your children are watching—and learning—from what you do. That includes your behavior in and near the water. It also includes your behavior after you've had a drink or two.

Shape. As we discussed, it takes time and practice to shape your children to understand and follow rules. At fun and active outdoor settings such as beaches and swimming pools, the shaping process is doubly important, and also doubly challenging. Work at it. Be consistent, firm, and disciplined about your rules. Reward safe behavior, and engage with your children. A parent who is in the water playing with her child will have more success than one who looks up from a magazine to yell at an unruly child across the swimming pool.

What Should I Do in the Neighborhood?

Children in the early school years are not safe traveling the streets alone. Period. The American Academy of Pediatrics suggests children should not walk across streets alone until age ten. Published research from my laboratory suggests we might train seven- and eight-year-olds to be safe pedestrians, but only with a good bit of time and effort. Scholars debate whether five- and six-year-olds can ever be safe pedestrians, no matter how much training they get or how smart they are.

So follow the TAMS method: start teaching, start shaping with rules (including "don't cross streets alone"), and certainly model safe behavior yourself. But the *A* in TAMS points to supervision near traffic, and that is an absolute must for children in this age group.

An adult must supervise children between five and eight years old carefully if they are in or near traffic.

Beyond facing traffic, there may be other risks in the neighborhood: climbing trees, risky behavior on playgrounds, swimming in open water, stray dogs, ice-skating or playing on thin ice, and more. The list could go on and on. How does a parent cope as his children gain increasing independence to wander neighborhoods alone or with friends?

Through TAMS, of course. Remember that you have shaped your child to behave safely, modeled safe behavior to her, and created a culture of safety in your home. Those lessons, which can be reinforced constantly through your modeling and shaping, will help your child make the right decisions as she grows older.

Concluding Thoughts

Parents' joy from seeing their children grow is unending, and the early school years represent a period of sustained physical, mental, and social growth for children. Savor these changes, and be proud in watching your child learn about the world.

As you witness your child's growth, always stay conscious of how you can build the desired culture of safety in your household. Model safe behaviors when you are together as a family, and seize opportunities to teach your child what actions you are taking to keep yourself and your family safe. Teach rules, and enforce them by commenting on positive and safe behaviors whenever possible.

Only when needed, discipline your child for unsafe behaviors. Remember that your children are growing and learning. They will make mistakes, and they will make poor decisions. This is the natural process of children becoming adults, and we adults must be forgiving and understanding, constantly conscious of the fact that children's brains work differently than our adult brains. These differences sometimes create risk for the child, but we can mitigate that risk through TAMS. Remember also that a firm warning is usually sufficient to motivate change toward safety. Then you can immediately redirect and move on to more positive activities.

Of course, beyond teaching, modeling, and shaping, you will also continue to act to protect your child's safety. Supervision and safeguarding do not disappear as your child grows. Let's close with a happy anecdote from Chelsea about how the TAMS method helped keep her eight-year-old twins and their friend safe.

We live in the city but spend a lot of time out at the farmhouse in the country. Ever since they were little, my twin boys have loved driving the ATV on the farm. They know the strict rules: helmet on, one driver only without passengers, stay on the paths, stay off the county highway, and drive slowly. Sometimes they argue over who drives first and who takes too long with his turn, but usually they do pretty well with it.

Last weekend they had a friend, Sam, come out to the country with us. Sam had never driven an ATV before, but he wanted to try. I honestly think most boys would have broken the rules—either had their friend ride as a passenger or let their friend try operating the ATV without telling me, or something else dangerous. But my boys did the right thing. They came to ask me whether they could teach Sam to drive the ATV. I guess I trained my boys well; they were shaped into being cautious.

We talked it over, and we agreed (at my suggestion, of course) that it would be hard to teach Sam to operate the ATV safely in just one afternoon. Plus his mom might not want him to drive it. Instead we agreed to let Sam drive the golf cart. I got in the front seat next to Sam, and the boys rode in the back. Sam drove the golf cart all over our property. We all had a great time, and we found a safe solution to the dilemma.

—Chelsea, mom of twin boys, age eight

Chelsea might need to reconsider whether her own boys are capable of operating the ATV safely (most experts would suggest they are too young). But beyond that detail, she clearly raised her twin boys well. They knew to seek adult help, overcome peer pressure, and avoid injury risk to their friend.

7

THE LATER ELEMENTARY SCHOOL YEARS

Ages 9–12

WOW, YOUR CHILD IS GROWING UP. Reaching double digits in age, making new friends, learning a lot in school, and probably engaged in one (or many) activities, such as sports, music, Scouting, and so on. Let's talk about how all that development might affect safety, and then review specific steps you can take to keep your child safe during these later elementary school years.

Cognition

Brain development doesn't slow down as your child grows through the later elementary school years. Your child is learning to consider, process, and act on increasingly complex tasks and situations.

Think about crossing a street as an example. Imagine your daughter is walking to a friend's house. The friend lives on the next street over in your neighborhood. Every neighborhood is a little different, but let's suppose your daughter is at a location where she has to cross a two-lane street, with one lane of traffic moving in each direction. She's at a mid-block crosswalk, not an intersection, and the traffic is moderately heavy. There are certainly times when she could get across safely, but it will take some patience to watch traffic and wait for a safe gap to cross between the oncoming traffic in each direction.

To get across the street safely, what sorts of things does your daughter (or any pedestrian, for that matter) need to do? First, she needs to look left, perceive the closest car approaching, and consider how far away that car is, how fast it is traveling, and whether it is accelerating or decelerating.* Inclines, curves, speed bumps, and other potentially relevant factors might be computed mentally also.

Once information about the oncoming car from the left is processed, your daughter needs to look to the right and process the same information: where the closest vehicle is, how far away it is, how fast it is traveling, whether its speed is constant or changing, and so on. Boy, this is a lot of information to process, isn't it? And it all has to happen very quickly because if there are delays, the cars will no longer be where she perceived them to be.

And we're not finished yet. Along with processing information about the two oncoming cars, your daughter also has to look across the road and figure out how far that distance is, and how fast she can get across each lane of traffic. So we've got to think about the distances and speeds of two oncoming vehicles, plus the distance and speed with which we can move across the crosswalk. If we delay in processing all this information—suppose it takes us a second or so—then the cars are closer, and our safety is jeopardized.

Is crossing the street easy? No. It takes a lot for a child's brain to do all this work, and the latest scientific research suggests that it

---

* If you happen to live in the UK, Australia, Japan, or another location where traffic travels on the right, just reverse the rights and lefts in this description.

may not be until age 14, on average, that typical children accomplish this task the same way adults do. When we add in more complexities—extra lanes of traffic, parked cars or shrubbery impeding vision, or (heaven forbid) a distracting smartphone—the risk of child pedestrians being struck by oncoming vehicles might increase.

The bottom line is that children's brains are still developing through the late elementary school years (and, in fact, well into the adolescent and young adult years). Complex cognitive tasks such as crossing a street must be conducted with caution. Your child may assume she has adult-like capacities, but that assumption is likely misguided. You must continue to function in your parent and adult roles to protect your child's safety through the TAMS strategies.

Social Influences

The TAMS method emphasizes modeling. We parents might engage in safe (or risky) behaviors, and our children will learn to act in similar ways. We discussed the research demonstrating the power of this mechanism for safe behavior, as in the examples of wearing seat belts and bicycle helmets. Children behave the way their parents behave.

As your child grows older, he is likely to model not just the behavior of trusted adults like you but also the behavior of others, including peers and celebrities. Consider Mia's story about her son, Xavier:

> My son, Xavier, has always been active. He loves to be outside, and he loves to be moving around all the time. I don't mind that. My husband is the same way, and it's good sometimes for boys to be boys. Over the last year or two, Xavier has gotten more and more into skateboarding. We bought him a new board for his birthday last year, and he absolutely loves it. He usually goes down to the local park and hangs out with his

buddies there. They go up and down the ramps and do tricks and listen to music, and it all seems like good, healthy fun. Xavier tells me he wears his helmet whenever he rides, and I trust him on that. We've taught him well about using safety gear.

One afternoon, I was busy preparing dinner, and I got a phone call. Well, *the* phone call. The dreaded one. A local police officer called and told me he was with my son at the park, and Xavier had a serious injury. The officer had called the paramedics, and the ambulance would be delivering my injured son directly to the children's hospital. The officer suggested I meet them at the children's hospital emergency department as soon as I could.

Well, of course I dropped everything in the kitchen and called my husband out on the golf course, and we both rushed to the children's hospital. When wo got thoro, thcy told mc Xaviçr waз being moved directly to surgery. He had a serious broken arm. The doctors called it an open fracture, which meant the bone had broken through his skin, and there was a high risk of infection. The good news is that it would heal. It wasn't a threat to his long-term health. The bad news is that it required surgery to repair, and he'd be in a cast for weeks.

That was bad news, but I honestly feared it might be worse. I took a deep breath and hugged my husband. A few days later, as Xavier started to heal, I asked him what happened. He remembered only some fuzzy details about his injury, but he also told me which of his friends were at the park that day, and I talked to them too.

I want to share the story with you. It started with Xavier's friend Carter. Carter was watching a YouTube video on how to do a really tough skateboard trick, the Willy grind. I never heard of this, but let me try to explain based on what I now know. The kids were actually at the baseball field and skating down a hill, then jumping with their board onto the first row of the metal bleachers by the field. They would then glide down the bleachers on the bottom of the skateboard—the wooden part, without using the wheels—and then jump back onto the ground to land on the wheels. Carter said it was a really tough trick. Sounded ridiculous to me!

Anyway, Carter had been practicing this Willy grind trick for a few days, and all the kids were watching examples of it on YouTube. Xavier was scared to try it at first, which made me happy to learn, but of course he was seeing a lot of his friends try it, and he saw all the YouTubers do it easily. So he gave it a shot. He was wearing his helmet, but he slipped, fell, and ended up with the serious broken arm.

Did I do something wrong? I'm not sure. Xavier is too old for me to be watching him constantly. I taught him well, and he was wearing his helmet. He also was a bit cautious apparently—he let Carter and some other friends try first. Of course, the end result is still this serious injury and weeks in a cast. What should I have done different? I'm not sure.

—Mia, mom of Xavier, age 11

Xavier's story is common. Peer pressures, modeling of celebrities and online videos, and a desire to fit in all influence children's behavior as they gain independence from their parents and engage in the world on their own. With alarming frequency, these influences lead to risky behavior.

What should parents like Mia do? Let's return to TAMS. We want children to act in safe ways, even if we're not there. Remember that it is healthy for parents to let their children explore the world independently as they grow older, just as Mia allowed Xavier to skateboard with his friends at the park. As Mia said, we can't watch over them forever. We also want to create that culture of safety in our household. To do that, we rely on the *T* (teach), *M* (model), and *S* (shape) portions of TAMS so that our children *A* (act) safely on their own.

We can teach our children lessons throughout their childhood. This teaching should start early and can continue as they approach adolescence and beyond. In Xavier's case, Mia could teach Xavier to always wear his helmet (this apparently was a successful lesson) and to learn new tricks carefully, in a step-by-step fashion. She could also teach Xavier to be sure he only tries tricks that are within his physical ability to complete (this apparently was not entirely successful). There may be safe ways for Xavier to learn the Willy grind step-by-step. Or he may need to recognize the Willy grind is just too advanced for his skateboarding skills, and he should have learned alternative tricks first, working up to the challenging Willy grind in the months and years to come.

We parents must also model safety. Few parents out there are passionate skateboarders, but behavioral science suggests modeling generalizes from one behavior to another. So if Mia were to model safe driving, safe bicycling, or even safe hoop-shooting in the driveway, then Xavier would likely generalize those decisions and actions to his own behavior while skateboarding.

Finally, we need to shape safe behavior. Our teaching and modeling will help accomplish this goal, but parents also can shape through other strategies. Mia might find a time, for example, to accompany Xavier to the park and learn about his skateboarding. To avoid embarrassment, this might be scheduled when other boys aren't there. Xavier can show Mia his tricks. She can respond mostly with praise, congratulating him on his skateboarding ability and—important—on how he is engaging in safe behaviors. If Mia identifies risks, she can point them out. This is a key part of shaping, but such admonitions should be balanced with ample praise and encouragement to achieve maximum efficacy.

What Should I Do in the Kitchen?

Some kids love to cook, and there are plenty of tasks even preschoolers can help with in the kitchen. By the later elementary school years, children are ready to start tackling complex recipes and meals, but risks abound. In particular, parents may continue to worry about the risks of cuts, burns, and fires.

My advice is to walk a fine line between teaching, demonstrating, and supervising until your child shows he can use potentially dangerous equipment safely. Most youth this age can learn to use knives, ovens, and stovetops safely, but you also need them to be prepared to handle unexpected situations. What if the vegetable slips while he's cutting it? What if the oil splashes into her face? What if the pan in the oven is heavier than expected? Will your child respond appropriately and safely? Or is there risk? Proper parental teaching, acting (supervising), modeling, and shaping will preserve your child's safety while learning to enjoy the joys of cooking.

What Should I Do in the Bathroom? On the Stairway?

Your child should generally be safe in the bathroom by this age, though we should mention a few minor risks.

Be careful of slips and falls. Wet floors and kids in a rush ("Get to school on time!") sometimes create a bad mix. At this age your child may also be using electric toothbrushes, hairdryers, or other bathroom devices. Children might also charge their omnipresent phones or tablets in the bathroom. Avoid electric shock risks: be sure your child knows not to handle electric devices with wet hands and not to use electric devices while sitting in a bathtub. Check that your home has ground-fault circuit interrupter (GFCI) electrical outlets in the bathroom.

Stairways offer another easy one at this age. Risk of falls down the stairs decreases dramatically as your child gets older. Continue to keep the stairs clear of debris, though. And consistently enforce household rules to prevent running, jumping, and horseplay on stairways.

What Should I Do in the Whole House?

As your child grows older, you are likely to leave her alone for longer periods of time. You might even leave her alone in the house for a short time (though many state laws officially prohibit doing this before age 13). Being alone increases the risk of children discovering, experimenting, and playing with dangerous items in the house—think about medications, firearms, knives, power tools, and so on.

Most of us assume our child would never play with a power drill, handgun, or container full of pills. In fact, most of us are correct. But a few of us are sadly wrong. Children die every day from accidental gunshot wounds and overdoses. And it's not easy to predict who will be right and who will be wrong. Most everyone thinks it will not happen to them, and most everyone is actually vulnerable. So take precautions to prevent a disaster. Follow TAMS.

Let's consider Tyler's story about his daughter, Holly, as an example:

Holly is in fifth grade. She goes to a good school and does well in her classes. She plays soccer, takes violin lessons, and dances in the local ballet studio. She's a Junior Girl Scout too, and she's awfully good at selling those Girl Scout Cookies each year. She's really an all-American girl in many ways.

Up until this year, we've always had birthday parties for Holly at community places, and she invited all the girls in her class. We tried the trampoline park, the bowling alley, the video arcade, and so on. Everyone seemed to have fun. This year, for her 12th birthday, Holly wanted to do something different. She wanted to just invite her three closest friends and have a sleepover at our house. I guess that's another sign of her growing up. My wife and I talked it over, and we agreed this would be fine. It actually seemed easier for us to plan.

The big day finally arrived. Holly's friends got to our house midafternoon and immediately retreated into Holly's bedroom. We checked on them every now and then. They were just giggling away, singing along with music videos, gossiping about the boys in their class, and so on. It all seemed like harmless fun. We gave them some snacks for an appetizer and then had a big pizza dinner, followed by birthday cake. They watched a Disney movie after dinner and then decided to watch a second movie. All seemed fine, and everyone was having fun.

Around 11:00 PM we sent the girls to bed. They all brought sleeping bags, and they were all planning to sleep together on the carpeted floor of Holly's room. They kept talking and giggling, of course, but they stayed pretty quiet, and we figured they would eventually fall asleep. My wife and I went to sleep too.

About 3:00 AM, I heard commotion. Seems the girls were up and talking, almost yelling. The voices were muffled, but I sensed something might be wrong. I dragged myself out of bed, threw on a bathrobe, and walked into the kitchen. I couldn't believe it! There were several bottles out on the kitchen table: orange juice, Coke, Sprite. They were in various states of emptiness. There was the sugar bowl I use for my coffee, a bottle of honey, and even a jug of milk.

And then there were three other bottles: vodka, rum, and whiskey. They were mostly empty, especially the vodka.

Uh-oh. Those bottles were mostly full last night. In fact, I think the vodka bottle was brand new. My wife and I don't really drink all that much, but our liquor cabinet has the usual stuff, and we do drink it occasionally. I couldn't believe the girls had gotten into it. It was also clear they didn't know what they were doing. Four preteens drinking most of a bottle of vodka, half a bottle of rum, and a touch of whiskey? They were surely very drunk, and in trouble.

I quickly located the girls in the bathroom, where at least one of them was vomiting. Sure enough, they were all very drunk. It seems they had drunk the liquor very quickly, so they were rapidly becoming drunk and sick. They were completely clueless, randomly mixing sweet drinks and downing them like Gatorade after a soccer game. Who knows what exactly they had put into their bodies?

I immediately woke my wife up. We piled all four girls into the minivan and drove them straight to the hospital. My wife made the tough calls, informing the other parents in the middle of the night. They met us at the hospital emergency department.

From there a lot of the evening is a blur. I don't even know exactly what the ER doctors did. I remember them talking about pumping stomachs, inserting breathing tubes, and giving IV fluids. I'm not sure. We'll be investigated by the legal authorities, and the other parents must be incensed at us. They should be. How did it happen? We let those four girls drink a bottle of vodka in our house? At our daughter's 12th birthday party? Seems impossible. But sure enough, it happened.

—Tyler, dad of Holly, age 12

Tyler's story is alarming. Alcohol poisoning can be very serious and even fatal. It also seems like the type of story many of us might possibly imagine happening to us. Curious and naive preteens get their hands on alcohol, medications, firearms, power tools, and any number of other dangerous items in the home. They experiment, often cluelessly, and get themselves into trouble.

Let's place this into the context of TAMS. Action, in the form of safe storage, is your first step. Cabinets that children can't access without an adult (or a key the adult has) are sensible and affordable. Supervision is also key, although not always feasible with this age group.

Modeling gets tricky. It might be easier for things such as firearms and power tools. In those cases we can model safe behavior, teach safety rules and the use of safety equipment, and then supervise carefully as the child learns. With alcohol, modeling may involve consuming wisely and refraining from behaviors such as binge drinking and drunk driving. With medications, perhaps consumption can be conducted privately, away from your children.

Teaching children about drugs and alcohol should not be overlooked either. Keep your lessons age appropriate, but teach your children what you do, and what they may want to do as they grow to the age when drinking alcohol is appropriate. Holly and her friends were clearly too young to be drinking alcohol, but if they had ever learned that vodka and rum are normally consumed in small volumes and over several hours, rather than in large volumes over several minutes, their condition may have been reduced to an inappropriate tipsiness rather than potentially fatal alcohol poisoning.

Finally, as we have discussed for most child injury situations, long-term shaping is important throughout children's development. Help your child learn to protect himself—to stop and think, take risky activities slowly, and think before acting.

What Should I Do in the Yard?

As your child grows older, she may be ready to help with yard work: gardening, mowing, and so on. That's great! It's an opportunity for learning, bonding, and assisting the family. But take caution: sharp tools can injure. Follow the TAMS method to teach, supervise, model, and shape safe behavior patterns. See the discussion in chapter 8 for more information about safety with garden tools such as lawnmowers and hedge cutters.

We've discussed the risk of swimming for younger children. By the later elementary school ages, many children are quite adept swimmers. Does this mean you can leave your child alone in the pool? Or leave a group of strong child swimmers together to watch each other?

The strong and indisputable answer is no. Consistent adult supervision and monitoring is needed; the risks are too great and consequences too severe in and near swimming areas. Swimming areas are a location where the TAMS method applies, but it might be capitalized as *tAms*—the action of an adult supervisor must supersede all teaching, modeling, and shaping that occurs.

What Should I Do in the Neighborhood?

As your child grows older, your child is likely to venture farther in the neighborhood to visit friends, shops, parks, and the like. This activity might frighten you, but it is generally healthy for your child. Exploring the broader world, gaining independence to reach destinations, making small purchases, and encountering new sights and sounds are all positive experiences as a child grows into an adolescent.

Of course, independent exploration of the neighborhood involves risk too. Traffic might be foremost in your mind. There are drunk drivers, distracted drivers, and just plain crazy drivers out there, and your child is vulnerable as a pedestrian or bicyclist.

The American Academy of Pediatrics suggests most children are safe in traffic by age 10. You can help prepare your child for traffic situations through the TAMS method:

- Teach traffic safety, starting at a young age and continuing through these older child years. Be opportunistic. Even during mundane times such as crossing a parking lot to the supermarket to pick up a gallon of milk, you can say something like, "Wow, that car is driving awfully fast for a parking lot. Sure need to stay alert near traffic these days, don't we?"
- Act by supervising when and where possible, and ensuring safety gear such as bicycle helmets are used.
- Model safe behavior when you engage with traffic as a pedestrian, bicyclist, or motorist.
- Shape your child's safety consciousness, starting at a young age and continuing to adulthood. Keep rule enforcement consistent,

even as your child grows older and even if she is a bit recalcitrant against those rules at times.

Other neighborhood risks parallel those at younger ages: playgrounds, tree climbing, stray dogs, swimming holes, and so on. Apply TAMS so your child stays safe while exploring and enjoying the neighborhood.

Concluding Thoughts

The principles to help an older elementary school child stay safe are quite similar to those used when that child was a toddler. Follow TAMS to create a household culture of safety even as your growing child gains independence to make her own decisions, associates with peers who may or may not be positive influences, and is increasingly exposed to risk-taking examples from the Internet and other media sources.

In fact, the TAMS method—especially the lessons you have taught and modeled, and the child you have shaped—becomes increasingly important as your child gets older. Here's why. When a three-year-old does something risky, such as climb up and get ready to jump off the top of a playground structure, it's likely that a parent is supervising that child and can intervene. The parent may yell, "Get down!" and avert the injury-producing jump. When an 11-year-old does the same thing, however, it's less likely that a parent will be supervising. That 11-year-old might be at the park alone, or with friends, and is going to make the decision on his own. If he has been taught and shaped to think before acting, he may get on top of the structure, realize it's awfully high, and then climb down safely (even if that means enduring some jabs from friends). If he has not been taught rules and shaped into safety consciousness, the result may be an urgent trip to the hospital's emergency department.

Thinking Ahead: Cars, Drugs, Alcohol, and More

Before we move on to discuss situations that span all child age groups, I'll offer one more piece of advice. Your elementary school student will quickly grow into a middle schooler and then a high schooler. Puberty, adolescence, and the teenage years bring on new challenges for parents and new safety risks for youth (think first about the big ones: teen driving and exposure to drugs and alcohol). A wise parent will recognize that not too much has changed, however. And don't worry: TAMS works for teens too.

When your cute little boy or girl grows into a hormone-laden teenager, remember that he or she is still your little boy or girl. He will grow more and more independent from you. She will make safety-related decisions on her own. Will she drive too fast? Will he drink and drive (or bike, boat, hunt, or otherwise engage in risky activities requiring sobriety)? Will she skateboard without a helmet? The list goes on, and our parental nerves feel like they might explode.

Remember, though, that you have implemented TAMS. This is where your effort to shape your child really pays off. She has learned the lessons she needs to be safe. He has learned to make the right decisions. Like all teens, your son or daughter might make a bad decision now and then, but remember that you have raised your child in a healthy way. Through TAMS you have created a culture of safety that will persist through the adolescent years and beyond.

PART III

SAFETY
FOR CHILDREN
OF ALL AGES

———

8

SPECIAL SITUATIONS

Risks That Cross All Age Groups

BY NOW YOU HAVE A GOOD SENSE of how TAMS works, why accidents are not really accidental, and how you can make a difference to create a culture of safety and prevent catastrophe in your family. You probably have already started making changes too. Perhaps you are supervising your preschooler more carefully on the playground, installing cabinet locks in your master bathroom, or teaching your third-grader to use the toaster oven safely.

In this chapter we'll consider some special circumstances in which safety is paramount for children of all ages, and how you can apply TAMS to reduce the risk in your family.

Sports

Sports and athletics are healthy for children. Whether it is soccer, golf, ballet, or karate, the physical activity, camaraderie and teamwork, and lessons about rules are all healthy outcomes.

Of course, sport also involves risk for injury. Think about the last time you watched professional football, soccer, or basketball. Surely the players experienced injuries, often minor but occasionally quite serious. Don't assume youth athletes are immune. An American Academy of Pediatrics report suggests youth soccer players may experience about three injuries per 1,000 hours of playing. Indulge me with a little math. Suppose your child plays soccer for four hours each week, two 14-week seasons each year, plus attends three weeks of summer soccer camp. In that scenario your child has about a 15 percent chance of experiencing an injury each year. Computing precise probabilities gets complicated here, but that's roughly 50-50 odds of an injury over a four-year period.

And don't assume girls are immune compared to boys. Research suggests that girl soccer players actually experience eight injuries for every seven injuries boy soccer players suffer. Girls are particularly vulnerable to certain types of injuries, including concussions and knee injuries, probably due to physiological differences.

One last warning. You may be thinking, *OK, I agree. Turned ankles, bumps and bruises. That's normal for athletes, and they'll recover quickly. They're young.* You're right. Most sports injuries are minor, but many youth sports teams experience at least one or two injuries each season that are serious enough to require the child's family to visit a doctor, and for the child to miss a week or more of competition. It's very possible your child will be one of those children sooner or later.

So how do you raise kids who choose safety in sport? Are the accidents just part of the game? No, of course not. Some injuries emerge from overuse—children who repeatedly engage in the same action (throwing a baseball, jumping to hit volleyballs, or any number of other actions) experience risk of injury. The solutions here are simple: cross-train and rest. We often want our children to specialize in a particular sport and watch them become true masters at that sport. This is probably fine in high school and beyond, but there is strong research to suggest younger children might benefit, both emotionally and physically, from rotating across different sports, trying different ones that involve different motions, and having some days to rest growing bones, muscles, ligaments, and tendons.*

Other sports injuries, and probably the ones you thought about first, come from the action of the sport. Most often they involve contact between two or more players, between players and stable objects (such as soccer goals), or between players and moving objects (such as balls, bats, sticks, clubs, or rackets). The TAMS method can help avoid these injuries through two pathways.

First, protective gear is necessary. Whether it is shin guards for the soccer forward, helmets for the hockey goalie, or chest protectors for the softball pitcher, youth must be taught to wear protective equipment consistently and always—at practices and games, during pickup matches in the park and in championship matches in the university stadium. The rest of TAMS is key too. Adults must model use of safety equipment. When Coach goes out to warm up the little league pitcher, that coach should wear a face mask. And adults must take action to prevent youth from engaging in sport without the required protective equipment. Parents, coaches, and referees must be firm in their insistence on protective gear.

Second, we must heed the rules of the games. Illegal play can lead to injury, and youth must learn to play aggressively—which often helps win in games like soccer, basketball, and lacrosse—but also legally, maintaining safety for oneself and one's opponents. Referees and umpires must be firm, and coaches must support even the strictest referee who maintains safety as a top priority.

---

* A side note on this point: overuse injuries don't arise only from sport. There is evidence that child musicians can develop overuse injuries from repeated motions on instruments ranging from violins to drums. Computer users can develop overuse injuries too. These might come from playing video games or writing blogs all day. So be aware, and encourage your child to try multiple different activities to avoid overusing muscles in just one.

One last point: this discussion falls in this chapter about children of all ages for a reason. We can and should shape children's safety in sport from a very young age. Those three-year-old T-ballers, ballerinas, and soccer players are undeniably cute as they run the bases backward or clumsily twirl in their adorable tutus, but they are also at an age where we can and must begin preaching safety as part of their engagement in sport. Don't be lax with the youngest children just because you think they are unlikely to get hurt. Instead view their young age as an opportunity to shape their awareness and consciousness of safety in preparation for their movement toward powerful home run trots, graceful grand jetés, and masterful corner kicks in the coming decade or two.

In the Car

Most of us live in a driving culture, which means you'll be driving your children around town to an extent that may sometimes make you feel more like a chauffeur than a parent. Car crashes are among the leading causes of child injury and death, and there's plenty we can do to keep our children (and ourselves) safe in the car.

Of course, one aspect of safety means driving safely: no distracted driving, no drunk driving, following traffic laws, and so on. This invokes modeling. We teach our children, future drivers themselves, to be safe vehicle operators. This also reduces adult injuries by avoiding crashes. But since our focus is on children, let's discuss the issues specific to children in cars.

At the top of our list is the car seat. Here's a not-too-publicized factoid: *Around 85 percent of car seats on American roads are installed incorrectly.* Yes, that's right: just about everyone has their car seat installed wrong. It's possible you're one of those rare 15 percent exceptions, but the odds are that you have an issue with your car-seat installation that could be fixed. It might jiggle a little left and right, or front and back. The straps may be too low or too high on your child's chest. The car seat might be damaged, on recall, or installed near an airbag.

So what's a parent to do? Let's first invoke the *A* in TAMS: *act*. If you're like me, the manual that came with your car seat is lost or tossed. And even if you have it, it may not do much good; it takes a lot of time to read, follow, and understand.

Luckily there are certified car seat technicians who can help. These individuals are trained and certified by organizations such as Safe Kids Worldwide, and they have expertise to help install just about any car seat in any car. If you do some online searching, you'll discover who they are and what events they conduct in your local area. At those events you can set an appointment and get expert advice, usually at no cost, to ensure your car seat is installed properly and learn to do it yourself.

As children grow older, they progress from one car seat to another, from reverse facing to forward facing, and eventually to a booster seat. Then they move to a regular seat belt in the back seat and finally a regular seat belt in the front seat. Those transitions—rear facing to forward facing to booster to back-seat seat belt to front-seat seat belt—baffle most parents. There's good evidence that parents tend to move their children to the next level too soon.

Solution? Movement to the next stage depends on your child's age, weight, and height as well as local laws. Car seat technicians can help best. Otherwise follow online guidelines from reputable sources, such as Safe Kids Worldwide, the Centers for Disease Control and Prevention (CDC), or your state government.

I want to mention two more risks in the car. First, we all know distraction from your phone is dangerous, but what about distraction from your child? There's research evidence to suggest adults who are conversing in a moving car will pause their conversation when the driver has a difficult maneuver to make—say, a lane change or a tight left turn. The adult passenger recognizes the driver's need to focus and naturally pauses the conversation.

But your toddler won't do that. He might be talking to you, crying, demanding food, or fighting with his older sibling. Stop and think! You are driving, and your child's demands, important as they may be, need to wait. Pull over to a safe place to resolve the food, bathroom, or squabble issue. This is one rare time when your focus needs to be on something else—safe driving—and not on your child.

Second, let's talk briefly about hot-car deaths, or heatstroke. You may remember hearing a story in the local news about this situation. It's a hot day, and somehow a parent leaves his baby or toddler in her car seat, forgetting she is there. The parent goes to work or shop, and the car, like all cars during a hot day, heats up quickly. The child dies of dehydration and heatstroke.

You may be thinking, *That would never happen to me. There must be something going on with those parents. I would never forget my child is with me.* Believe it or not, that's what most victims of this terrible situation also say. Most incidents occur when there is some unusual change in schedules. Mom has a morning dental appointment, so Dad is taking the child to daycare and drives to work instead out of habit. Or Dad has an early meeting at work, so Mom is in charge of the childcare drop-off.

Habits are hard to break, so we automatically drive to our normal morning destination. The best solution to avoid hot-car deaths is to create a new habit. Leave something you will never forget—perhaps a phone, purse, or briefcase—in the back seat of your car, near your child. When you reach your destination, you'll remember both the phone *and* your child (plus, as a bonus, this trick removes distracted-driving temptation too). Another idea is to play children's music in your car while you drive, instead of your normal preference. That might lead you to engage with your child by singing along with the songs or having a conversation if your child is old enough. Even if your child is still very small, tell him what you are seeing as you drive. Hearing language and interacting with parents is great for children at any age.

Lawns, Gardens, and Farms

Gardening is a terrific hobby. Watching a tomato plant grow, flower, and fruit, and then enjoying the homegrown taste, is a true pleasure for child and parent alike.

Lawn mowing (and associated tasks like edging and shearing hedges) is often a drudgery but a necessary homeowner chore.

Farming is, for many, a living. It's often hard work, but also enjoyable at times, and involves long hours and physical demands.

Gardening, lawn mowing, and farming are very different in some ways, but from a safety perspective they have parallels. They involve tools, blades, and machines that were built for use by adults. They require physically demanding, often repetitive tasks that can lead to careless and distracted behavior. They are also tasks frequently delegated to children, even if children may not have the capacity or training to do them safely.

Let's pause on that last point. Gardening, lawn mowing, and farming are sometimes delegated to children, but those children may not have the capacity or training to complete the assigned tasks safely. TAMS can help us. Consider June's story:

My husband and I both grew up on a farm, and we love living on our beautiful two-acre plot out in the country. But there are drawbacks. One of those drawbacks is mowing the grass. Even with our new riding mower, it takes a few hours. It's a tough job on a hot summer day.

Since Tex turned 12 this spring, my husband and I decided he was old enough to operate the lawn mower. We knew his work might not be perfect—he may miss some corners or whatever—but we figured he was old enough to get the job done adequately, and it would save us parents time in our busy schedules. Plus Tex sits around and plays video games half the summer. Mowing would get him off his behind and doing something productive. We even paid him a few dollars to do the work.

The weekend after school ended, my husband went out and taught Tex how to use the lawn mower. The training lesson was pretty long and detailed, and Tex seemed to pick up on how to do it quickly. He's a smart kid, and he's usually pretty careful too. It went great for the first few weeks, but then the tragedy occurred.

For some reason Tex agreed to let his younger sister, Cass, ride along while he mowed the yard. Cass was just five years old—too young to be anywhere near that mower. But she sat on Tex's lap as they cruised up and down the yard. I don't know exactly what happened, but somehow, as Tex made a turn to start the next row, he hit a bump and Cass fell off the mower. Her arm got caught under the blades.

Tex came running and yelling. I saw Cass, and her arm was all blood. I called 911 immediately, and luckily the fire station isn't too far down the county highway. They took Cass straight to the hospital in town. The news was bad. The doctors had to amputate Cass's arm just below her elbow. They couldn't save it. Tex won't be mowing anymore for a while. And our family will never be the same.

—June, mom of Tex, age 12, and Cass, age 5

Tex was trained to drive the mower, but he wasn't old enough to handle all the potential risks of mowing. In most instances, 12-year-olds are not old enough to operate a riding mower safely.

To figure out when your child might be able to safely engage in a particular task, check online for the Cultivate Safety guidelines (https://cultivatesafety.org/) I helped create about gardening, lawn mowing, and agricultural tasks for children. In June's case, wise action and shaping about rules would have been a better choice, rather than trying to teach and model a complex task that Tex wasn't yet ready to handle safely.

In other cases, children can learn to garden, mow, and farm safely. Even young school-age children can begin to pick weeds and remove rocks from growing plots. Small backyard gardens or single fruit trees invite supervised picking of the fruit by young children.

As children grow older, chores can intensify. Move to sharp blades with caution, only after ample teaching and modeling, and with intense supervision initially. Move to machines with blades—such as a riding mower—only when children are well into their teenage years.

Firearms

Firearms. Guns. Weapons. Just the thought of those words rings all sorts of bells and alarms. Some of us are fearful: we'd never keep a gun in the house and hope our children never touch one. Others of us are excited: we enjoy hunting or shooting and teach our children safe handling of firearms from the time they are toddlers.

There's no right answer, and political opinions aside, a few facts are clear:

1. Most children in the United States are exposed to firearms in one way or another.
2. Firearms can be extremely dangerous if stored or used improperly.
3. Children can learn to hunt and shoot safely, and to enjoy hunting and shooting, if families choose this path and children are properly trained.

Whichever path your family chooses, TAMS can guide you. If your family decides guns will be off limits to your child, then you can teach and shape your child with rules that fit your family. These might include "Always stay away from guns," "Never touch a gun," and "If you see a gun, tell a trusted adult." You can also model such behavior.

If your family decides your children will learn to use firearms, then TAMS will guide you to teach safety, model safety, act safely, and shape your child to respect the power of a firearm. You or other trusted adults will supervise your child as she learns to enjoy hunting and/or shooting, and you will teach your child basic rules, such as "Always keep your finger off the trigger until you are ready to shoot," "Never point a gun toward another person," and "If you hold or see a firearm, always assume it might be loaded." If you keep firearms in your home, you will compulsively and constantly store them safely. With proper application of TAMS and attention to both the joys and dangers of firearms, you and your family can derive great pleasure from hunting and shooting sports if you choose to do so.

One other parenting challenge regarding firearms occurs outside your own home. What do you do about firearms safety when your child visits other people's homes? Whether it's a playdate or a visit to Grandma and Grandpa's house, how do you investigate and then handle firearm safety for your child in someone else's home?

The answer to that question varies across scenarios and based on your child's age and firearms safety training. No matter what, TAMS helps. For young children, you as a parent need to act. Ask the playdate's parents if they have firearms at home and how they are stored. Insist on safe storage if firearms are present. If you know your in-laws hunt, be sure their rifles are properly stored before your holiday visit.

For older children, and especially older children who have firearms safety training and experience, your long-term teaching, modeling, and shaping will kick into gear when they visit homes with firearms present. Your children have learned what to do when they encounter a firearm and how to behave safely so they are not hurt.

When You Travel

Whether it's a weekend getaway to a nearby state park, a week at Disney, or three weeks exploring European capitals, travel with your children can be extremely rewarding. It can also be extremely disruptive to your daily schedules, creating all sorts of risks for injury. Let's talk about the risks while traveling first, and then we can move into the prevention strategies.

Perhaps the best way to think about the risks while traveling is to imagine yourself on vacation. What constitutes a vacation will differ for each person or family, but there are a few key commonalities. First, there is risk of parent distraction. You may be enjoying the beautiful views of nature, lounging on the beach, or reading commentary about artifacts at a museum, but in all cases your attention may be taken away from your child.

Second, there is risk of fatigue. You're sleeping in a new bed and a new setting, as are your children. You may be in a different time zone or observing later bedtimes. Sleepiness and fatigue lead to different child behaviors, and different adult behaviors. Risks can emerge.

Third, especially for parents of young children, you're likely in a location that has not been safeguarded the way your own home has been. Cabinets may be unlocked, stairs ungated, and outlets uncovered. Whether it's Grandma's house or a Holiday Inn, new risks abound, and children may discover them.

Given these risks and others you may have imagined, what can you do to reduce risk? Short-term solutions are not too difficult. They represent strategies you enact while you are traveling. Following the TAMS method, supervision is essential. You may be easily distracted in a new and exciting setting, but so is your child. Keep alert and watch your children, of all ages, carefully.

To supervise your child best, stay engaged with him. Look at beautiful nature and museum artifacts together. Visit child-friendly destinations such as zoos, science museums, and even local playgrounds. Slow down, discover, and sightsee. Remember, this is a vacation! Spend time together. Your child will grow up fast, so relish these quiet moments of reflection away from the stresses of home and work.

There may also be ways to safeguard your environment while traveling. These will not be the same as you have at home, so don't neglect supervision duties. But if you have young children, consider ways to reduce risks, such as moving hotel furniture to block electrical outlets or readjusting the placement of corkscrews or glasses that young children could encounter.

If you're near water, remember the grave risks of drowning. At the beach, lake, or swimming pool, keep a close eye on your children. Don't allow your smartphone, a magazine, or a quick snooze to distract you from supervisory duties.

Vacations often involve walking near traffic. You might cross parking lots to a breakfast restaurant or busy thoroughfares to a glorious beach. Keep an eye out. Excited children may make impulsive mistakes near traffic. Calm adults should apply TAMS to reduce risk through teaching, acting, modeling, and shaping.

And finally, don't forget car safety! Use car or booster seats that match your child's age and size, and install them carefully in rental cars or Granddad's sedan.

Longer-term solutions for vacation safety build on the overarching goals of TAMS. The teaching, modeling, and shaping you have done for many years, and will continue to do for many years, must continue. These steps will yield a household culture of safety through repeated application, even on vacation.

Thus, family rules should be maintained. A special afternoon ice cream treat is fine, but expectations and compliance to safety rules should continue at all times, even at a vacation resort. Diligence to those rules is a key part of shaping and will yield consistent safety-conscious behaviors among all parties at all times.

Your modeling is also important. Don't lax up just because you're away; to the contrary, be consistent in your safe engagement with the settings you encounter. Practice safety on the water, in traffic, and at the park. Remember always that your child is watching you. Your behaviors are being observed and learned.

And last, have fun! Vacations are joyful family occasions that will yield a lifetime of memories. Staying safety conscious should reinforce your enjoyment, not disrupt it.

House Fires

Just the thought of a fire in your home is scary. Here are five simple actions you can take to reduce risk:

1. Act and model. Make sure you have smoke detectors installed and that they are functioning, with working batteries. These low-cost devices will alert and awaken you in case of a fire. Get them installed, and check them regularly. This is a mostly passive injury prevention strategy. Once you do it, it's done. And it saves lives.

2. Act. Hire an electrician to check your home's grounding. If lightning hits your home, will the charge carry through your house to the ground?

3. Act, teach, and model. Avoid overloading electrical outlets or using extension cords. Electricians can help with this problem too—spend the money to keep your home safe from electrical fires.

4. Act and model. If you use a woodburning fireplace, be sure it is inspected regularly and that the fireplace and chimney are confirmed safe by a professional.

5. Plan ahead. Know what you will do in case of a fire. Remember also that children sleep much more deeply than adults. That's their biological predisposition. Guess what that means? You may hear a smoke alarm at night, but they may not. Plan with your

partner who will awaken the children, how you will escape the house (and a backup plan if your first escape route is blocked by smoke or flames), and where you will meet to account for everyone's safety once you're safely outside the home. Plan also in advance who will call 911.

There's no getting around the fact that house fires are scary, and it's emotionally difficult to plan for scary events that are unlikely to occur. But planning ahead could save your child's life, so take the effort and reduce the risk.

9

A WALK THROUGH THE CALENDAR

Child Safety During Holidays and Celebrations

———

OH, THE SPLENDID thought of holidays. Delicious food and drink, joyous laughter with family and friends, needed respite from work obligations, and memories to last a lifetime. Historians document the celebration of holidays back to ancient times, perhaps starting with recognition of astronomical events such as the winter solstice. In today's world, many of us celebrate with our children soon after birth. These celebrations include both religious milestones such as baptisms and brises and secular celebrations such as Halloween trick-or-treating and birthday parties.

How do all these holidays affect children's safety? Negatively, I'm afraid. Research from several different countries and cultures all reaches the same conclusion: child injury rates increase during national holidays. This is true in summer and in winter, with religious and nonreligious holidays, and for kids of all ages.

Let's take a walk through the calendar, consider the child injury risks that emerge throughout the year, and then plan the steps you can take to prevent them.

New Year's, Thanksgiving, and Other Indoor Family Holidays

What better place to start the calendar than New Year's Day? As adults we might associate New Year's Eve with a glass of champagne and a loved one's kiss, the kids safely tucked into bed.

After a short night's sleep, the first morning of the new year is welcomed with family. Parades march, football games kick off, and tired parents enjoy time together to eat, drink, and relax with the family.

Where are the children, though? Remember TAMS. Who is actively supervising the kids on New Year's Day? Are we modeling safe behavior? Teaching safe play?

Other winter holidays that are celebrated indoors present similar situations and raise similar questions. Consider this story from Beverly, who was celebrating Thanksgiving with her large family:

Thanksgiving has always been a big holiday celebration in my family. My brother and sister and their families, my parents, and sometimes even some of the in-laws all get together in one place. My siblings and I rotate who hosts the dinner, so every three years the party is at our house. This year it was our turn.

Along with my husband and I and our three kids, we had 13 guests: my sister and her family, my brother and his family, his wife's parents, and of course our parents, who are now in their early 70s. Cooking a Thanksgiving meal for 18 is a lot of work! I did have plenty of help in the kitchen, and most everyone brought a few side dishes, but it's still a lot of work.

It probably won't surprise you that thinking about the kids' safety was pretty low on my priority list that afternoon. There were 10 adults in the house; surely they could manage the 8 kids. Plus a few of the kids are already teenagers, and we're past the baby stage. My sister's youngest is four years old now—no little tiny ones to worry about anymore.

Well, it's hard to put together exactly what went wrong, but here's what we know. I was working in the kitchen with the moms and grandmas. We were scrambling to chop, wash, prep, and cook. The dads and granddads, plus the two teenagers, were watching football in the den. Not sure how much it matters, but apparently the Cowboys were in a tight game and had just scored a beautiful touchdown.

Downstairs in the basement, the six younger children were playing. That's my own two younger ones (nine-year-old Brett and six-year-old Julie-Anne), my sister's two (five-year-old Alexis and four-year-old James), and my brother's two younger ones (eleven-year-old John and eight-year-old Melissa). It seems like Brett and John, the older boys, were playing the board game Battleship in the corner of the basement. The three girls, Julie-Anne, Alexis, and Melissa, were playing dress-up with some dolls in a different corner.

That left four-year-old James alone to explore the basement. He probably wasn't much interested in the dolls, and it was fun to explore all the toys and games in his cousins' basement. Apparently he discovered a kit of Brett's that is supposed to let kids do metalworking and woodworking. He pulled the box down from a shelf and poured out all the various tools and instruments. The kit had things like kid-friendly hammers and screwdrivers and glue, plus various metal and wood pieces. Not ideal for an unsupervised four-year-old.

All of a sudden, the older boys say they heard crackling noises. They looked up from their game and saw James lying flat on his back gasping for air. He wasn't breathing right at all, they say. The electrical outlet was charred, and James's fingers and hand were all black and burned. A toy screwdriver was lying on the ground, also charred.

The older boys dashed upstairs to alert us adults, and we all dashed back downstairs. What a scary situation! Luckily my brother's mother-in-law is a retired nurse. She attended to James and assured us that James's breathing was stabilized. His heart rate was OK too. We carried him up the stairs to the car and rushed him to the emergency room. The doctors there treated the burns on his hand and evaluated for internal damage.

Needless to say, the Thanksgiving turkey was burned, and dinner wasn't so festive this year. We picked up fast food on the way home from the hospital.

—Beverly, mom of Julie-Anne, age 6,
Brett, age 9, and Liam, age 13

Beverly and her family had a rough Thanksgiving celebration, and they were lucky that James survived with only burns to his hands. Let's break down what went wrong.

If we consider the situation from the TAMS perspective, a failure for Beverly and the other adults to *act* for safety is the most glaring hole. During a holiday, failure to act is understandable but inexcusable. Holidays represent our own downtime, an opportunity to relax and socialize with family and friends. The men surely enjoyed watching the Cowboys game together. Much as they were working hard to prepare the meal, the women enjoyed camaraderie in the kitchen. It was easy to assume the kids were safe on their own in the basement, especially with the older boys (ages 9 and 11) present.

Of course, the situation was not safe. No adult was supervising four-year-old James or the other young children. The older boys had not been told to keep a close eye on James or to include him in their activities. Even if they had been told to supervise their younger siblings and cousins, they would have been appropriate supervisors for only a few minutes, not a few hours.

Instead the adults should have worked out a way to keep a close eye on the children. They could have rotated to take turns in the basement, they could have kept the youngest children upstairs near the kitchen or den, or a few of them could have taken the group of children out to a park to play safely. Leaving the group of young children alone in the basement was a risky mistake.

The adults also failed to act by safeguarding the basement. Electrical outlet covers are inexpensive and easy to install. Age-appropriate toys might have been left for James and the other young children, with toys designed for older children removed temporarily to a safer location. Safeguarding a room for a one-day holiday celebration may seem excessive, but when it prevents a potentially fatal electrocution injury to a four-year-old, the safeguarding may suddenly feel like a good idea.

Independence Day and Other Outdoor Family Holidays

As the yearly calendar progresses and the weather turns warmer, holiday celebrations tend to move outdoors. Thanksgiving banquets and New Year's Eve galas are replaced by picnics and barbecues. Board games and dress-up dolls in the basement are replaced by swimming pools and yard sports. The risks for child injury and the need to enact the TAMS method remain omnipresent, however.

In fact, many of the holiday risks that are present during indoor celebrations are the same when we move outdoors. Action occurs through adult supervision and safeguarding of the environment. When you safeguard an outdoor environment, remember the biggest risks. Secure fence gates outside swimming pools and hot tubs, and properly store risky outdoor items such as tools, fuels, and gardening shears.

Shaping and modeling must continue during the warm-weather holidays too. Safety rules remain in place, whether it's a holiday or not. Continued and concerted effort should be devoted to rewarding safe behavior, even when we're socializing with family or distracted by festivities.

Summer holiday celebrations may even offer unique occasions to teach children about safety. Consider this story from Bill, whose family traditions led to an excellent opportunity to teach children about safety with fire:

I live out in the country and work as a volunteer firefighter while holding down my day job in home construction. We have a tradition in our family to build a big bonfire in the yard on the Sunday night of Labor Day weekend. I've been doing this for years now.

In the bachelor days, it always turned into a huge bash. After Candy and I got married, we toned it down a touch, but it was still a full-day affair to build the bonfire, light it around dusk, and then party the evening away with a large group of friends and family. We continued that tradition after the kids were born, hiring a babysitter to watch the kids indoors while we celebrated with an adults-only party out in the yard.

Now that the kids are getting older, it's time to think about some more changes. All our friends have kids too, and it seems like it makes sense to upgrade the Labor Day bonfire celebration to a family event. Of course, I want to do so carefully. Some of the kids are still pretty young, and I've seen the horrible results of young children and fires in my work as a firefighter. With a load of kids surrounding a big bonfire, we have to think carefully to avoid any accidents.

Candy and I discussed how to do this safely. We decided to go ahead and change the Labor Day bonfire to a family event, with three major changes to assure safety.

First, we knew we couldn't abandon the idea of a bonfire. That was the heart of the tradition, but we needed to set it up to make sure no kids would get close to the fire. So I built the bonfire like normal, but then I put a ring of rocks and logs around the bonfire, at a pretty good distance—probably 15 feet or so. That ring marked where you could go. No kids were allowed past the ring of rocks and logs. Only me and a few other adults (my fellow volunteer firefighters) were allowed to go past it, and that was only to tend the fire and make sure it was burning safely. I told all the parents about this safety ring when I invited them to the bonfire, and we reminded everyone when they arrived. Everyone liked that plan.

Second, we knew we didn't want kids running around unsupervised and bored. We asked all parents to watch their own children at all times. They could still socialize with each other, but parents were responsible for their own children and were required to watch them at all times.

Third, to keep both kids and parents entertained, we set up stations all over the property. These stations gave kids fun games and activities to do, and parents could talk while they supervised kids at each station. We hired a group of high schoolers to work at the stations and give kids little prizes after each one. It was set up kind of like a carnival, really, so the kids would have activities to try, and the parents could talk to other parents as they traveled from one station to the next.

Some of the stations had food and drink available. Several of them had basic outdoor games like cornhole, lawn bowling, and sack races. But given my work in fighting fires, I also wanted to use the bonfire tradition to begin to teach kids, including my own kids, about safety with fire. So we set up two stations to specifically teach children about fires and fire safety. I chose the most mature high schoolers, who had babysitting experience, to run these stations. Plus parents were always with their children and closely supervised at both these stations.

One of those stations was a small firepit where the kids could roast marshmallows. That let them get close to a fire and see how hot it was. The two high schoolers working at this station gave the children careful instructions about how the fire was hot and dangerous, and how they could use a long stick to roast their marshmallow, but they had to stay far away from the fire. That was especially nice for the younger children.

The other station was better for the older children at the bonfire. We set up a long row of candles on an old dining table I had out in the garage, and the station was designed to teach children how to light candles. We had both matches and lighters available for kids to try. It's amazing how many of the kids had never lit a match or a lighter! They would light the candle, let it burn for a few seconds, and then blow it out. I was stunned how much the kids enjoyed this activity. It was a hit of the party, almost as big a hit as the huge bonfire! And they learned how to safely light and blow out fires.

As it is every year, the Labor Day bonfire tradition was a great success. Given those memories of the early Labor Day bonfire years, it was a little bittersweet to revise it to a family event. And the party definitely ended earlier in the evening this time around. But we made the right decision. And the new format was a huge success. Both parents and children loved it and said they looked forward to returning next year. We had no accidents with the fires (or anything else). And we managed to teach all the kids something about fire safety in the process.

—Bill, dad of three children, ages 4, 7, and 11

Bill and Candy demonstrated creativity and resourcefulness, and their efforts paid off well. They hosted a safe and successful outdoor holiday celebration. They assured careful supervision by the parents attending, they supported supervision through safeguarding of the bonfire with a ring around it, and they supplemented those strategies by hiring high schoolers to run each station. Bill's clever ideas to teach children about fire with the marshmallow firepit and the candle-lighting table are impressive and worth replicating in your home. And everyone, young and old, enjoyed a family holiday tradition without injury.

Before we move forward in the calendar to autumn holidays, let's discuss one more aspect of outdoor holiday celebrations: fireworks. Here in the United States, we almost universally associate fireworks with the July 4 Independence Day holiday. In other countries fireworks are similarly associated with holidays: the Lunar New Year in China, Bastille Day in France, the Diwali festival in India, Eid al-Adha in predominantly Muslim nations around the world, and Christmas in much of Central and South America.

It's not surprising that fireworks-related injuries to children are common around those holidays. In fact, around 70 percent of the fireworks-related injuries in the United States happen during the July 4 holiday season. Each summer several thousand children suffer serious fireworks accidents. Many suffer eye injuries that lead to blindness. Others suffer hand and arm injuries that lead to amputations.

To avoid fireworks injuries to children, it's best to let adults—and sober adults, at that—do all the lighting and setting off of fireworks. Children can watch but not light.

Alternatively, go to professional fireworks displays rather than lighting fireworks at home. If children insist on participating, give them poppers or sparklers that pose much less risk, and supervise carefully.

Take care, though: fireworks injuries peak in early July, but they represent only a small portion of the many injuries children experience. In fact, almost all injuries to children during the July 4 holiday are *not* fireworks injuries. Instead they are the same types of injuries that occur all the rest of the year: car crashes, drownings, poisonings, falls, and burns. Your solution is natural by now. Implement the TAMS method to prevent all types of injuries, including fireworks-related ones. Teach, act, model, and shape to create a household culture of safety while still enjoying holiday celebrations.

Halloween

Halloween is one of my favorite holidays of the year. That's probably because I'm both a parent and a child psychologist.

Halloween is such a kid-friendly holiday. The simple act of dressing in costume is inherently tied to youthfulness, allowing us to pretend we are someone else and engage in the childlike fantasy of otherness. We parents enjoy the glee in children's faces as they wander the streets in costume, yelling "trick or treat" to complete strangers and receiving candy treats as a reward. What a cooperative tradition—a community joins together to provide happiness for our children.

I am often approached by journalists during the Halloween season who ask me what injury risks might be elevated for children during the holiday. We might think first about risks in treats that have been tampered with. Will our child bite into an apple that has a razor blade hidden inside? Will children wolf down a candy bar that was unwrapped, unknowingly ingesting poison along with the sugary treat? These are slight risks, and parents should inspect their children's treats to toss anything that is unwrapped, but these risks are really rather small.

The bigger risks come from walking the streets. Trick-or-treating often occurs after dark. Sometimes children are unaccompanied by adults. Sometimes children's vision to see traffic is occluded by masks or costumes. And most alarming, sometimes the drivers are intoxicated or distracted, forgetting that they must take special care that evening with youngsters wandering the streets.

Parents should counteract those risks through TAMS. Help your children choose costumes that allow them to see well. Supervise them as they walk their neighborhoods. And consider whether light-colored costumes, reflective strips, or carrying a flashlight might make sense.

Other risks are also present. Carving pumpkins together presents an opportunity to teach or model knife safety. Younger children might draw faces on their jack-o'-lanterns with markers, rather than carving them.

And don't forget that candy is a choking hazard for young children. Find appropriate treats for young children. Go ahead and gobble up the rest yourself!

Christmas, Hanukkah, and Other Gift-Giving Holidays

Where does one begin when thinking about the December holiday season? Religious, cultural, and family traditions vary, but almost all children eagerly await tasty treats, uplifting holiday music, a break from school, and the opening of presents. We parents celebrate also. Enjoy the happiness and joy of the season as you make merry and build family holiday traditions.

We also know the holiday season can be stressful. Stress leads to lapses in safety. TAMS reminds us to return to the basics, and that message emerges ever so clearly during a hectic and busy time like the December holidays. You can avoid lapses in teaching, acting, modeling, and shaping safety during the distractions of the season through diligence and habit. Continue to model safety, even when stressed or rushed. Continue to shape behavior with consistent rules and expectations, even when children are out of school. Act with safe supervision, even if children are playing outside during chilly weather or playing inside because it is too cold to go out. And find opportunities to teach safety, especially by involving children in holiday-related activities such as cooking family recipes, lighting holiday candles, and hanging holiday lights and decorations.

The gift-giving tradition of Christmas, Hanukkah, and other holidays deserves special attention. Step 1 for safety is selecting the right gifts for your children. Pay attention to the recommended age listings on the gifts you select. In many cases those age guidelines are carefully determined by government officials who make their decisions based on child safety. Such guidelines should be observed; giving a young child a gift that is designed for use by older children can lead to serious injury risks.

Step 2 is to examine the gifts your child receives from others. Even if you carefully scrutinize each of your own purchases at the toy store, Auntie Jane may recklessly select the first recommendation she sees online, without considering potential safety hazards. So after your child rips open the wrapping and screams with delight, do a quick scan for product safety. Is your child ready for this gift? If Auntie Jane goofed, don't ignore the situation. Calmly and firmly tell your child that you are putting Auntie Jane's gift away to play with later, and store it until your child grows into the safe age group for it.

Step 3, the last step, is to use gift-opening time as an opportunity to practice TAMS. The mad rush to open presents under the tree on Christmas morning is among the most precious and special times in a child's life, so it may seem difficult to interrupt through TAMS strategies. Consider how Nikki did it, and think about whether a similar strategy might work in your household:

It's Christmastime again, and the kids are excited as ever. It seems as if we have more presents under the tree this year than ever before. Perhaps I went a little overboard at the mall—not sure. And my mom always piles the gifts high for her grandkids.

Anyway, at about 8:00 AM on Christmas, everyone was awake, and the kids were literally drooling over the pile of presents. I got my phone out to take photos and let them have at it. Jesse is the oldest at age eight. He showed his little sisters what to do. Find your pile, rip the paper off, scream in delight, and repeat. Continue on and on until your pile is gone. If we parents are lucky, perhaps a thank-you here and there.

Jasmine is five, and she seemed to know what she was doing also. She and her older brother attacked with delight. Jade is just three, but she quickly figured out how to rip paper off her gifts. And she certainly knew her way around screaming in delight when she got to those doll babies. Wow, was she excited!

Well, the stacks were getting lower, and soon Jesse and Jasmine were both finished. Jade was a bit slower. When she reached her last present, she was stuck. It was a box that had been shipped with her name on it, but it wasn't actually wrapped. I think it was from my brother, who ordered something online and had it shipped here to our house directly. Jade knew she had to use scissors to open that one, and Jesse had already retrieved scissors from the study to open his packages.

So Jade grabbed the scissors in her fist and started poking at the box, trying to break the taped seals. I looked over and saw her flailing wildly with the scissors in her fisted hand. "No, stop!" I yelled amid the hubbub. Everyone looked up. Jade started crying. I was worried, though. She could easily have poked her leg or arm with those scissors, and she clearly didn't know how to use them. She also was never going to get the package opened that way. She knew I was mad at her, and I hated to see her cry on Christmas morning, but I also didn't want to be taking her to the ER with a scissors blade sticking out of her thigh.

After the initial moment, Jesse and Jasmine went right back to their new gifts. My husband started helping Jasmine put together some sort of building kit she got, and I took a deep breath, remembered TAMS, and got down on the floor to hold Jade and calm her down. I knew what I had to do: teach her how to use scissors, and model safe scissors use too. I showed her the best way to open a package like this and let her "help" me by holding my hand as I did the cutting. We finally got the package open, and it was a beautiful little toy piano. She was happy again and started banging away on the piano. I was glad I could implement TAMS and teach Jade about scissors safety, even in the craziness of Christmas morning.

As I reflected on the situation, I realized I probably should have implemented other parts of TAMS. I might have anticipated this issue and gotten some child-safe scissors out the night before from the kids' playroom so all three kids were using blunt and safe scissors rather than the pointy adult scissors Jesse found in the nearby study. I also could have dealt with the package for Jade better. It had been so hectic the last several days that when the package arrived, I just threw it under the tree. But it might have been smart to open up the package myself after Jade was asleep and wrap the gift in paper. That would have avoided the whole problem of needing scissors in the first place. Guess I'll try to remember that for next year.

—Nikki, mom of Jesse, age eight,
Jasmine, age five, and Jade, age three

Nikki was a role model for implementing TAMS in the heat of the moment, a moment with emotional excitement that may surpass almost any other time in the year. She also illustrates to us the value of reflection. She used TAMS to handle the immediate situation beautifully and then reflected further on the situation later, recognizing steps she could take to implement TAMS and reduce risk in the future.

Whether your family's tradition is hanging ornaments on the Christmas tree with grandparents, chanting blessings while lighting menorah candles, singing traditional melodies while drumming the beat, or visiting the mall while wearing ugly (but beautifully coordinated) sweaters, enjoy the holiday season. But remember to do so safely. Implement TAMS, spend quality and loving time with your children, and take steps to assure they will learn to continue your family traditions safely someday with their own children and families.

Birthday Celebrations

Once a year, a special holiday occurs. Birthdays are particularly special for children because their birthday is their own holiday, a special day unique to themselves (twins and multiples excepted, of course). Families tend to celebrate this uniqueness by granting the birthday child special privileges—perhaps she selects a restaurant for a family breakfast together, decides what clothes everyone in the family will wear that day, or chooses the scrumptious dinner that is served at home that evening. In most families the day is also celebrated with a birthday cake and presents.

The specialness does not occur just at home either. Many schools make birthdays special for children, allowing them to host a small party with their classmates or wear a special crown, badge, or sticker to designate the specialness of the birthday.

Despite all this uniqueness, which should be celebrated and enjoyed, safety cannot be compromised. Parents should maintain TAMS and never neglect the need to shape, model, teach and act. Don't neglect supervision after new presents are opened. Use birthday candle lighting and cake cutting to model or teach fire and knife safety, respectively.

Children's birthdays are also celebrated with parties. The classic picture of yesteryear involved a few classmates over to your house after school for cake, ice cream, and backyard games. That picture has evolved to today's habit of weekend gatherings with large numbers of children at specific birthday party locations such as skating rinks, crafts shops, and video game parlors. This raises all sorts of challenges for parents, who must work to maintain the safety of not only their own children but also all their invited guests. Consider this story from Lynette, who had a party for her 11-year-old at a local trampoline park:

Whenever our kids have a birthday, my husband and I throw a big party for their whole class. We've tried climbing walls, laser tag, bowling alleys, and skating rinks. This year my daughter Olivia wanted to try the new trampoline and inflatables park for her 11th birthday. An hour of jumping up and down—not for me, but I know the kids love it. Plus it's just down the street from our house, so I was happy to go with Olivia's suggestion.

We booked the party and e-mailed out invitations. It was pretty standard for a birthday party package: the kids get an hour to run and play in all the trampolines and inflatables, and then you get a party room for

30 minutes to serve drinks, cake, and ice cream. Their staff helps manage everything with us parents, and all the kids seem to love it.

Olivia invited her whole class of 25, both the boys and the girls. My younger daughter, Sophia, would come along also, and we let her invite her closest friend so she wouldn't be left out.

Well, the big Saturday arrived. Olivia welcomed all her friends, and they set off into the jumping area. As the kids were playing, I worked to decorate the party room and make sure the cake, ice cream, and drinks were ready. I also set out the plates, napkins, cups, and silverware. My husband started to move all the birthday presents out to the car so Olivia could open them at home in the evening—no time to do that during our 30 minutes in the party room.

All of a sudden, one of the party staff people burst into the party room. She was really almost a kid herself—probably just 15 years old or so—and her face looked absolutely panicked. "Your daughter got hurt," she yelled. My heart started pounding. I worried, *What does that mean? Little bump to her leg? Major concussion?* As my mind was racing, I think I muttered something like, "OK, where is she?"

The staff person scurried out into the jumping area, and I nervously and quickly followed. As we got closer, I could hear a girl crying, and then I realized it wasn't Olivia who was hurt, it was Sophia. I don't know why I assumed it was Olivia; I guess probably because it was her birthday.

Anyway, I ran up to Sophia to see what was wrong. I went to hug her tight, and she reached out her hand and pushed me away. "My arm hurts too much!" she screamed in pain. Her right arm was kind of hanging limp, and she couldn't move it. I'm no medical expert, but I had to assume probably her arm was broken.

I didn't know where my husband was at this point, so I called his cell phone and told him where we were and what happened. We agreed to meet in the parking lot. I took Sophia with me and drove her right to the hospital. How ridiculous—I was driving my eight-year-old to the hospital in a car filled with her older sister's birthday presents. My husband stayed behind to handle the rest of the birthday party and then asked one of the other parents to deliver him and Olivia to the hospital on their way home.

> Turns out Sophia had a serious arm fracture. She was jumping on a trampoline with some of the older girls from Olivia's class and somehow fell off, breaking her arm in the process. It was terribly swollen by the time we got to the hospital, and she'll need a cast and sling for several weeks.
>
> —Lynette, mom of Olivia, age 11, and Sophia, age 8

Lynette's story might feel familiar to you. Trampolines and inflatables are an integral part of our children's lives these days. Much as they offer great fun and great exercise, they are also dangerous. What could Lynette have done differently? Let's think about the TAMS method, step by step.

Teach. Lynette didn't really talk about this, but she could have taught her children to behave cautiously in settings such as trampoline parks. Sophia probably would have been safer jumping only with her friend, who was younger, rather than trying to jump in the same area as Olivia's friends, who were three years older, and three years bigger.

Act. Many birthday party venues rely on young and inexperienced employees to supervise children. The party environment is typically safeguarded reasonably well, but child injuries still occur with alarming frequency. This is especially true with birthday party activities that involve some risk, such as trampolines and inflatables. In those settings there is great value in helping to supervise the children. After all, other parents are entrusting you (and the facility) to keep their children safe.

Consider the possibility of inviting other parents to stay for the party too. Ask them to help you supervise the children while they play, and reward them with a big piece of birthday cake afterward. Ask the facility to let you arrive early to set up and decorate the party room so you can devote your attention to supervising the children while they play.

Model. If Lynette is anything like me, she probably doesn't have frequent opportunities to model safe trampoline jumping with her children. However, she can model relevant lessons that would translate to her children, and so can you. Consider how you judge the limits of your physical abilities. Only attempt tasks you can safely complete. For example, when you drive, do you wait patiently at an intersection for a safe gap between oncoming cars to turn into, or do you slam down the accelerator to squeeze into a tight gap? Do children notice such behaviors and then replicate your patience (or impulsivity) in an inflatable obstacle course?

Consider also how you behave when you notice others engaging in health risks that could impact you. For example, what do you do when exposed to secondhand smoke? Do you move away to protect your own health? Might your child model this behavior when exposed to older and bigger children on a trampoline? Perhaps he would recognize his risk and move to a different trampoline with peers his own size.

Shape. As we've discussed, shaping is a long-term process, but one that offers substantial benefit to children when they engage in unfamiliar settings where emotions may be high, such as a birthday party. If you've shaped your children within a culture of household safety, they will likely display that safety everywhere, including while gleefully jumping on a trampoline with friends.

There's one more point to make about this story. It probably wasn't entirely a coincidence that Sophia got hurt instead of Olivia. She was young and playing on inflatables and trampolines with older children. But she was also *not* the birthday girl. Birthdays can be tough on siblings. All the attention is focused on the other sibling, and feelings of jealousy and neglect are commonplace. This can lead to attention-seeking or risk-taking behavior, and sometimes to injuries. We parents need to stay aware of such risks and be sure siblings get some attention as well as appropriate supervision during brother's or sister's special day.

Concluding Thoughts

One rainy day in the near future, take a look at your old photo albums. It doesn't matter how old the photos are or whether they are on paper or digital. Whatever you look at, you'll likely discover that many of our most precious memories are formed during holidays. How many of those special images in your photo album were snapped during holiday celebrations? A good number, I suspect.

For this reason, among others, you should enjoy holidays. Savor them. But create those memories within the context of a household culture of safety. Remember that most injury risks during the holidays are exactly the same as the risks during the rest of the year. Risk is elevated because we adults can be tired (late nights celebrating), distracted (busy cooking, entertaining, and socializing), and/or relaxed ("It's a holiday; the kids will be fine"). Don't allow fatigue, distraction, or complacency to interrupt safety. Maintain the TAMS method through the holiday just like you do any other time.

Do attend also to the special risks that emerge during holidays. A surprising number of those risks revolve around fire and burns—both religious and secular holidays are associated with lighting candles and fireworks. Just as Bill did at his Labor Day bonfire, use this as an opportunity to teach children about fire safety. And model safe behavior yourself. Consider carefully the child pedestrian risks on Halloween and kitchen safety on Thanksgiving.

Most important, celebrate. Holidays represent our escape from the daily grind. Enjoy time with your children and families, and take plenty of photos to fill the next pages in your album.

10

WHAT ABOUT WHEN THE KIDS ARE BEING WATCHED BY SOMEONE ELSE?

LOTS OF THINGS make us parents nervous, but high on the list are those first moments when we are separated from our child. The first day of preschool. The first sleepover. And sometime in the almost unimaginable but actually not too distant future, the first solo drive to high school.

This chapter helps us think through the safety of our child when we are not there to provide it directly. The solution may seem baffling at first. How can we possibly provide for our children's safety if we are not even physically there with them? The answer probably won't surprise you: turn to the TAMS method.

Remember, TAMS helps us establish safety in our household, and that safety extends to all settings and situations. We have taught our children the safety rules they are old enough to absorb. We have modeled safety. And we have shaped our children to engage safely in the world, to follow safety guidelines, and to demonstrate caution when there might be risk. With dedicated use of TAMS, you will create a culture of safety that does in fact keep your children safe even when you are not physically there with them. You will raise your kids to choose safety.

Regrettably TAMS may not solve another problem that may be lingering: your own anxiety and nerves. It's natural and normal for us parents to be nervous about our children's health and safety. We love them so deeply, and we can't fathom any harm ever coming to them.

In fact, just the act of seeing our children experience pain is hard for us parents. As an example, we dread the thought of our children's immunization shots. We know the shots are good for their long-term health, and we also know there is short and mild but temporary pain involved. For that reason, we loathe the trip to the pediatrician's office for annual shots.

Be warned, though! Scientific research suggests children rate themselves as experiencing much more pain during immunizations when their parents are nervous compared to when their parents treat the shots as a routine medical procedure involving what it truly is: a small and minor prick.

So what's the parenting message for injury prevention? Calm and relaxed parents have children who not only experience less pain when they get their annual shots but also negotiate the world with greater confidence and independence. They will also likely engage in the world more safely.

How can we parents relax our nerves and stay calm about our children's safety when they are outside our supervision? If you've consistently applied TAMS, your nerves should already be calmed. TAMS creates safety, even when you are not there. It may take some effort to process this reality, but you must convince yourself that your child is safer with TAMS in place. You taught him well. You modeled safety. And you shaped him into the child you want him to be: someone who explores and experiences the world to learn and grow without taking dangerous risks.

To understand this process better, let's consider a few common scenarios where you leave your child alone and may fear potential injury risk.

With the Babysitter

Leaving your children home with a babysitter can be nerve-racking. In many cases your child's supervisor is still a child herself; you're entrusting your child's safety and life to a teenager. And you're supposed to go out and have fun while you do that!

Understandably many parents struggle with this notion. They fail to enjoy themselves while they are out because they are worrying about what might be happening back at home. They constantly check their phone for messages while supposedly out having fun with their partner. Or they spend hours considering and selecting the best babysitter only to use him infrequently because it causes too much stress.

I can't provide you with all the solutions, but if you've applied TAMS in your house, there are plenty of positives to consider in the equation here. First, in most cases you've left your child at your own home, which you know is properly prepared to reduce risk because you engaged TAMS to safeguard your home. Second, you're probably not too far away. If there is an urgent situation, the babysitter has your phone number and can reach you quickly and easily. Third, and most important, you've created a household culture of safety. Your children will choose safety even if you are not there because you have been using TAMS. They have been shaped carefully. They know what they should and should not do. They know what they can and cannot play with. And they know they are being watched.

Let's repeat that last point: they know they are being watched, and by an authority figure. Even though that teenage babysitter may feel like a child to you, that same babysitter feels like an adult to your child. Think about it this way: from a 4-year-old's perspective, a 16-year-old teenager doesn't feel too different from a 26-year-old teacher, a 36-year-old mom, or a 66-year-old grandma. They are all adults with the authority to set and enforce rules about safety. And as we discussed back in chapter 6, they are all adults who will cause children to behave more cautiously because they know they are being watched. Quality supervision from a babysitter will yield safer behavior from your child.

While we're taking perspectives, let's also consider where the babysitter is coming from. You've surely hired that individual with care, working to identify a responsible and mature individual to watch over your children. That babysitter knows she is responsible for your child and is likely to be highly vigilant to avert any problems. She should be focused and dedicated to the task of keeping your children safe as a top priority, while also accomplishing secondary tasks such as entertaining your children, feeding them, and getting them to sleep on time.

There are a few additional steps you might take to reduce the risk of accidents occurring. Can you have dinner prepared in advance so the babysitter only needs to serve the meal, rather than becoming distracted from supervising in order to prepare it? Can you time your outing to minimize risk? Perhaps leave a touch later so your children are asleep for much of the time you are away? Could you send your oldest child to a friend's house for a sleepover, leaving only the younger one under the babysitter's care?

No matter what you do, remember that TAMS creates a situation in which parents can safely leave their children with others. You have taught and modeled safety. You have acted to safeguard your home and shaped your child amid your household culture of safety. You have hired a babysitter you expect to also be an appropriate teacher, actor, and modeler.

Think of it this way. There are times when parents need to take time to themselves without guilt or regret. Babysitters permit this respite. Whether it's supervision of your young children playing, daily chores such as laundry and dishes, or finding a moment to discuss household finances with your partner, life as a parent is busy and stressful. Take opportunities to relax and enjoy yourself. Don't fret over your child's safety. Your application of TAMS keeps your child safe when you're out.

With the Grandparents

There's a funny thing about parent-child relationships. They never end. No matter how old we are, Mom and Dad are still Mom and Dad. They will always be older than us, and therefore they will always have some amount of wisdom and experience that we lack. Even if it frustrates us at times, and even if we sometimes (or often) disagree, there is great value in considering our parents' perspectives as we implement parenting strategies with our own children. Take a moment to reflect upon how your parents raised you, and try to replicate the things that worked well. Encourage and allow your partner to do the same.

Taking it one step further, try this exercise from the TAMS perspective. Think about the parenting strategies you saw as a child and how they might fit into the TAMS model. Copy what worked.

Of course, the world changes, and we parents of young children have plenty of knowledge and experience that our own parents lack. I imagine you know your way around a smartphone better than your folks. You can navigate multiple streaming services, the smart doorbell, and the Uber app with ease, whereas your parents may be content with old-fashioned cable TV, push-button doorbell chimes, and hailing taxis from the sidewalk.

So how does all this influence our children's safety when we leave our kids with Mom and Dad, either our own or our partner's? Let's hear from Eva to consider the issues:

My husband, Jacob, works at a bank downtown. Every December his company has a holiday party, and it's pretty much mandatory for employees and their spouses to attend. The boss and the boss's boss and even the boss's boss's boss are there. It's at the fancy country club and really kind of annoying and artificial. But I guess it's part of the job to show your face, shake hands, and smile at the important people, so Jacob and I go every year.

Jacob's parents live near the country club, so we decided to skip the babysitter and drop Ella off at their house while we attended the event. Ella is 29 months old, almost two and a half now. Jacob's parents planned to take Ella to the park to play for an hour, feed her dinner, and then read her some bedtime stories. We brought the portable crib so they could put her to bed around eight thirty. We planned to pick Ella up after the work party ended and take her home to sleep the rest of the night back home.

Everything went as planned on our end. We dropped Ella off with the in-laws and went to the country club. Jacob introduced me to his new boss and we chatted with her for a few minutes. We shook hands with the boss's boss and exchanged pleasantries and happy holiday greetings with a bunch of Jacob's other coworkers. We even got our photo taken with Santa Claus! Dinner was fine; the wine was pretty good. Oh, and I bumped into an old high school classmate too. She wasn't a close friend back in the day, but it was a pleasant surprise to see her, and we enjoyed catching up after all these years. She has a two-year-old also, and it was fun to compare parenting notes.

When it seemed appropriate, we snuck out of the event and drove over to Jacob's parents. Ella was asleep as we expected, and we sat down for a few minutes to get a report on their evening. Seems they had fun at the park, and Ella really enjoyed watching the pigeons. They brought some old bread to feed the birds—what fun!

When it came time to hear about Ella's dinner, though, we got the biggest surprise of the evening. Let me try to replicate what Jacob's mom said. It went something like this:

"I wanted to make sure Ella was eating a healthy dinner, so we got those nice organic beef hot dogs. I gave her a hot dog without a bun and then some green grapes, mashed potatoes, and baby carrots on the side. I knew the carrots would be hard for her to chew, so I chopped them up into small pieces. Like you told us, we filled her sippy cup up with milk and then let her have a small piece of cheesecake for dessert. She ate really well and seemed to enjoy the food a lot.

There was one strange thing, though. The grapes seemed to be hard for her to eat. She coughed and spit them out once or twice, and we even had to bang on her back because she was having trouble swallowing them."

I didn't know what to say. I was in shock. I was happy they tried to give Ella healthy food, but how could they feed her grapes without cutting them into small pieces? Didn't they know Ella's throat is still very small, and grapes are a major choking hazard at this age? How could they not know that? I didn't even bother to ask about the hot dog, but I bet they didn't cut that up either. I was at a loss for words, and I was fuming mad.

Thankfully, Jacob jumped in. It's all a blur, so I don't know exactly what he said, but he somehow explained to his parents what they had done wrong and why certain foods, such as grapes, are a choking hazard to young children. I think probably Jacob's parents felt bad, and I'm sure they won't do this again. But it sure upset me.

We drove home in silence, and I went straight to bed.

—Eva, mom of Ella, age two

Eva had reason to be angry with her in-laws. They put Ella's life in danger by feeding her foods that present a choking hazard to young children. As parents it's hard to anticipate all the possible risks when we leave our kids with the grandparents, but reviewing the dinner menu beforehand may have helped Eva and Jacob avert this tragedy. They likely would have reminded Jacob's parents to cut the hog dog and grapes into small pieces if they knew that was the planned menu.

Beyond that, it takes patience and understanding to leave our children with the grandparents. If you ask about safeguarding the home, reducing choking risks, or most any other contemporary safety recommendation, they are likely to respond with some cliché response such as "Well, this is how I did it with you, and you turned out fine, didn't you?"

Your response to that catchphrase must be worded carefully, perhaps something like this: "Yes, but many other kids my age never grew to be parents themselves because they died of an accident. Think of how medical science is saving the lives of so many cancer patients these days. Safety devices such as car seats and smoke alarms are doing the same thing. Experts in injury prevention have figured out new ways to save children's lives, and even though you didn't use them when I was a kid, it's important to use them now. We know more, and we need to do everything we can to keep our kids safe from injury. I know you love your grandchildren; please help me keep them safe."

With careful wording, your parents are likely to learn a lesson from you. They will change their behavior.

Before we move on, I want to address one more tricky part of leaving your kids with the grandparents. How do you deal with the pills? In fact, this applies to leaving children in all sorts of places, but it emerges quite frequently at grandparents' homes because older people often take more prescription medicines. Rhoda explains:

It's June 6, the one-year anniversary of the saddest day in my life. And the five-year anniversary of my happiest day.

I can barely write about it.

Last year for our fourth wedding anniversary, Ted and I decided to have a date night. Just a nice dinner and a movie, nothing wild, but a nice opportunity to spend a quiet and intimate evening together without the kids. We put on some nice clothes, left the two kiddos with my mom for the evening, and planned to pick them up the next morning. Joey was two at the time, and Kelsey was just three months old.

From what I understand, Mom had her pill minder out on the coffee table, where she always keeps it. She was upstairs changing Kelsey's diaper and putting her down to sleep when it happened. Joey found Mom's pill minder and ate a bunch of the pills. I guess he thought it was candy or something.

When Mom got back downstairs and found the pill minder mostly empty, she was worried. She knew pills were missing, and Joey said he had eaten them. The details don't really matter, but Mom thought Joey was fine at first because he didn't show any symptoms. She kind of figured he would puke them out. Kelsey was sound asleep, and Mom didn't want to bother Ted and me during our anniversary dinner.

After Mom watched him for a while, Joey started to look really drowsy. Mom decided to call me. She figured our movie would be over by then. I asked what Joey's symptoms were, and Mom said he just looked tired. It was 9:30 PM at that point, well past his normal bedtime, so I told her to put him to bed and check on him before she turned in. I didn't realize what a mistake that was.

The next morning we went to pick up the kids around seven. Kelsey was already awake and looked great. I went upstairs to the guest room to get Joey, and there he was in bed. He looked like he was sound asleep, peacefully lying on his back. I tried to wake him up, and he didn't respond. He just lay there. He was cold and motionless. My two-year-old little boy was dead.

I shrieked. The rest is hard to write. The doctors said that Joey probably died because he ate a few of Mom's buprenorphine pills. That mixed with some of the other pills in a bad way. It probably caused Joey to stop breathing during his sleep.

—Rhoda, mom of Joey, deceased at age 2,
and Kelsey, now age 15 months

There's a saying among doctors: "One pill can kill." Sadly, Rhoda and her family learned that lesson.

Like many people grandparents may remove their pills from child-resistant containers and put them in pill minders or other contraptions to be sure they remember to take the right pills at the right time. This can work great when only adults are around.

When you place kids into the mix, however, you need pills to be stored safely, away from any location where kids might get their hands on them. You also need to supervise. I sometimes think of this as the 3 S's: Supervise and Store Safely.

This isn't always an easy conversation to have with your parents, but TAMS action is required. Be sure medications and any other risks to children are safely stored and inaccessible when your children visit their grandparents. And be sure supervision is consistent when safeguarding is imperfect.

At Playdates and Sleepovers

When you send your children to another parent's home, you may be on safer turf than when you send them to your parents' home. Other parents are usually of the same generation as you, they have children in the home already, and they probably read and follow safety guidelines like you do. Perhaps they even use aspects of TAMS. But that doesn't mean there aren't worries and concerns to consider.

Here's a story from Liz:

Cecil is eight years old now, and he was just invited to his first sleepover! I'm so excited for him, and he's excited too! The sleepover will be at his friend Luke's house this Saturday. They will play together for the afternoon, eat dinner, watch a movie, and then sleep overnight. I'll pick Cecil up Sunday morning.

It all seems so perfect, but there is one issue bothering me. You see, we've known Luke and his family for a few years now, and I fully trust them. They will take care of Cecil like he was their own son. From what I can tell, I agree with Luke's mom on just about everything parenting-wise, *except* one thing. And it's kind of a big thing. We are a no-guns household. I just don't want to have guns in the house where my kids might discover them. I know there are other perspectives, but that's the way I feel.

Luke's mom is different. One day when we were out on the sidelines of the boys' soccer game, the topic of guns came up. Luke's mom told me she keeps a pistol in her nightstand, just in case she needs it for self-defense. Her husband keeps one at his bedside too, right under the bed where he can grab it quickly if needed. And they have a gun case for all their hunting rifles and shotguns. I didn't really say anything that afternoon out on the soccer field; I just listened and nodded. I know there are a lot of people like them, and it didn't seem like the right place or time to disagree or start a discussion about such a sensitive topic.

But now my eight-year-old son is about to spend the night in their home, without me. I assume Luke's parents are pretty careful. I know they are good parents, and the guns are probably locked or unloaded or whatever is needed to keep them safe. I doubt Cecil would even go into Luke's parents' bedroom. But it still worries me. What if Cecil and Luke found a gun and started playing with it? What could happen? Maybe it's partly because I don't understand guns very well, but it scares me a lot.

I wasn't sure what to do, so I decided to turn to my sister for advice. She's always thoughtful about this kind of problem. Her recommendation was pretty clear: be open with Luke's family about your concern, and address it head-on.

My sister was right. I called up Luke's mom. I thanked her for having Cecil over for the sleepover and then expressed my concern about the guns in a friendly but firm manner. Luke's mom was understanding. She assured me almost all the firearms in the house were unloaded and locked, and stored with the ammunition in a different, safe location in the house. Her husband kept one pistol loaded by his bedside, just in case of an emergency, but that pistol was stored in a case that only opened with his fingerprint. They boys could not possibly access it.

But Luke's mom also said she would talk to her husband, and they would make adjustments to ease my nerves. They would double-check the safety of all the guns in the house before I dropped Cecil off, and she would put the unloaded gun she kept by her bedside into the gun case for the whole time Cecil was visiting. Her husband would unload his bedside pistol for the night and store the ammunition separately. The gun case would be locked up, and only Luke's dad has a key on him. The spare key is kept at Luke's grandparents' house. That way there was no way the boys could possibly discover a firearm and hurt themselves.

I was glad I took action. TAMS worked even though I wasn't even going to be there with Cecil. I called my sister for advice, and then called Luke's mom to discuss my concerns. I was happy with the outcome and appreciated Luke's mom's understanding. In the end, I kept my Cecil safe and created a situation that would let both him *and* me enjoy his very first sleepover without worries!

—Liz, mom of Cecil, age eight

Liz's story offers plenty of good lessons. First, sleepovers are healthy for children, and for parents. They allow children to grow and mature in a healthy and positive way, and they can be held safely by planful parents. Second, you can take steps to assure your child's safety when she goes for a sleepover or slumber party. Get to know the other parents, and assure yourself they are like-minded and concerned about children's health, safety, and well-being. Take action if you discover any concerns. Liz's story illustrates the *act* portion of TAMS marvelously.

Third, seek input from those you trust. Liz turned to her sister and received excellent advice. Think about your close personal network and whom you can turn to when you need advice and input to deliver on TAMS and assure safety for your child.

Let's also briefly consider the perspective of Luke's mom. She also applied TAMS, perhaps unknowingly. She and her husband kept guns in their house, but even before Cecil's visit, Luke's parents were meticulous about storing the firearms safely, in most cases unloaded and with ammunition in a separate, safe location. The loaded pistol by Luke's father's bedside was stored in a locked case that could be opened only with the father's fingerprint, in case of emergency. Luke's mom also responded well to Liz's concerns, showing empathy and identifying a compromise both families were comfortable with. Open and frank communication, in both directions, led to a fun sleepover for both kids and their families.

At Day Care and School

Many American day care centers and schools are routinely inspected and approved by licensing or accrediting bodies. Inspectors and auditors focus on the quality of education, of course, but they also incorporate into their reviews topics such as the safety of the school environment and injury risks for the children. Thus, if your child's day care center or school is licensed or accredited, you can be assured that a third-party agency has examined the school with at least some degree of detail attended to your child's safety.

With that said, injuries still occur in day care centers and schools. A huge portion of those injuries actually happen not inside the school building but on the playground. How can you keep your child safe when they are at school and away from your supervision?

If you've consistently practiced TAMS, your child will know how to keep himself safe. He will act as you have raised him through teaching, modeling, and shaping. He will make safe decisions and behave cautiously when there is risk. George's story shows TAMS in action.

I'm in sixth grade. This is the last year we get recess at school—once we get to the junior high, they give you short breaks but no recess. Bummer. Recess is my favorite part of the school day! I especially like playing kickball and touch football. Sometimes we boys get a little rough, but it's all in good fun.

Recently we've been playing tag. I don't like tag as much as the other games, but I play anyway because that's what everyone is doing. One problem with tag is that there are always fights about who is it. Who touched who? Does it count if you touch their shirt instead of their skin? Do you need two hands or just one? What if you touch them with your foot? The fights go on and on, and they take the fun out of the game.

Anyway, today Freddy got really mad. He said that he had tagged Ricardo on the hand, but Ricardo said he didn't feel anything. This happened right by the swing set, where the girls were talking, and Ricardo and Freddy started yelling really loud at each other. The teachers didn't seem to notice. They were standing way over on the other side of the playground, by the school building. All of a sudden, Freddy picked up a bunch of gravel from the area below the swings and threw it at Ricardo.

Ricardo was mad, so he picked up a bunch of gravel and threw it back at Freddy. The girls shrieked and ran away. Some of the boys ran toward Freddy and Ricardo and started throwing the gravel at each other too. I think most of them agreed with Ricardo and were throwing the rocks at Freddy, but a few seemed to be on the other side of the argument. From what I can tell, it was just a mass of about eight or ten boys throwing rocks at each other randomly, and a group of girls running away and yelling.

I stood still for a second and thought about what to do. I kind of agreed with Ricardo. From what I could see, Freddy didn't tag him, and

Freddy sort of has a tendency to lie sometimes. But I wasn't sure running into that gravel-throwing craziness was a good idea. Someone could get hit in the head and be hurt. Or what if a rock hit your eye? That could be really bad.

I turned around and—hate to admit it—followed the girls. Yes, I just ran away and toward the school building. At that point the teachers figured out what was going on and started yelling and blowing their whistles. They got it broken up pretty quick, and all the boys involved got in trouble. I think some of the parents even got called in for meetings with the principal. I'm glad I ran away. It was the right decision.

—George, age 12

George was right, of course. He made the safe decision to stay away from what some might see as "typical boy behavior." It seems pretty unlikely that anyone ever taught George not to throw rocks at other kids on the playground. It seems even more unlikely that his parents or any other adult ever modeled such behavior. Instead George was exposed to wise and safe decision-making. His parents surely deserve some credit there because they taught, modeled, and shaped George to make a good decision despite some peer pressure to engage in the risky behavior.

And one side point: George was also right to be concerned about eye injuries. Hundreds of thousands of children experience eye injuries each year, the most serious of which cause permanent blindness. Being struck by a rock in the eye could result in a very serious injury.

Concluding Thoughts

Leaving your child with others is understandably heart wrenching. In almost all cases, it is harmless; in fact, in many cases it allows your child to grow and mature. But that doesn't ease our fear of the unknown and our fear of the rare disaster.

The solution is twofold. First, practice TAMS. Help your child learn how to keep herself safe. By using TAMS, you are giving your child the tools she needs to make safe decisions and avoid injury, just as George demonstrated for us on the playground.

Second, take action. Act by choosing your child's supervisors carefully. Find the right babysitter, select the right school, and question sleepover hosts before leaving your child. Act also by ensuring safety. That's the lesson Eva and Jacob learned when they failed to double-check their daughter's dinner menu with Jacob's parents. It's also the lesson Liz learned when she approached Luke's parents to ask about firearms safety in their home. They are lessons you can easily adapt to the situations you face as a parent. Acting to create a safe environment and a culture of safety will ease your own mind as well as ensure your children's safety.

11

INJURY PREVENTION
FOR CHILDREN WITH
SPECIAL NEEDS

RAISING A CHILD WITH SPECIAL NEEDS introduces parenting challenges. The challenges vary widely depending on the child's needs but invariably involve extra time, effort, and commitment from loving parents.

When it comes to child safety, the influence of a disability can be equally varying. Consider the simple act of crossing a street safely. A child with a hearing disability may not hear traffic approaching. A child with attention-deficit / hyperactivity disorder (ADHD) might impulsively dart into the roadway, inattentive to the oncoming traffic. A child with an anxiety disorder may be fearful of crossing, hesitating on the sidewalk before entering the roadway and then entering the road with increased risk as the traffic gets closer. A child using crutches may cross the street slowly, increasing risk by staying in the roadway a longer time. The lesson is obvious: each disability creates different risks, and those risks might vary in each different situation.

There is one commonality across all children and all situations, however. Application of the TAMS method helps. All children can be taught, and all children can be shaped to engage safely with their world. All children model their parents' behavior too. And of course, we adults can take action to keep all children safe, no matter what their disability.

I want to make one key point first. The advice and ideas for children with one type of special need usually can be adapted to children with a different type of need. In fact, these ideas usually transfer easily to children without special needs as well. So don't worry if your particular situation doesn't quite fit. I recognize that every child is a bit different from every other child, and every parent is a bit different from every other parent. You will need to adjust the advice to your child and your situation, but if you adjust thoughtfully, you will achieve the desired culture of safety in your home.

Children with ADHD

ADHD is hallmarked by patterns of impulsivity, inattention, and/or hyperactivity. On the surface this might seem a true recipe for disaster when it comes to injury prevention. A child who is hyperactive might run and climb and jump all over the place, leading to injury risk. A child who is inattentive might not notice safety rules or cues. And impulsivity seems perhaps the biggest concern. A child who is impulsive will act without thinking, diving right into dangerous situations.

I've got some good news and some bad news. Let's start with the bad. That recipe of impulsivity, inattention, and hyperactivity does lead to increased risk for injury. Children with ADHD are hurt somewhat more often than children without ADHD.

The good news is that those trends are reversible. With application of the TAMS method, parents can keep children with ADHD safe from injuries. To do this, patient teaching and consistent modeling are essential. The need for shaping is also amplified, and parental action is especially important for young children with ADHD.

Let's consider Maya's story:

CJ has always been a wild little boy. Could never get him to sleep as an infant, threw his food all over the kitchen at age three, and don't even get me started about trying to keep him still and quiet at church. He seems to love only the park and playground, where he can run and play freely.

About a month after CJ started kindergarten this past fall, the teacher called my husband and me in for a meeting. She thought CJ might have ADHD and recommended we get him evaluated by a psychologist. We set an appointment, and the psychologist agreed with the teacher. CJ has ADHD.

We thought about starting him on some medicine to help, but he's only six years old. So we decided to try counseling first and see if that would be enough. CJ goes to counseling every week now, and it does seem to help.

One consequence of CJ's ADHD that hasn't gone away is that he always seems to be getting himself hurt. Scraped knees and elbows are practically a daily occurrence. We've had turned ankles, loose teeth, and even a wasp sting on the ear lobe! But today's story might be the best one yet.

CJ got out of school around 3:00 PM, and we went straight to the supermarket. It's funny: even though CJ is so active and always on the run, he still likes to ride in the shopping cart when we go to the supermarket. I guess he's still a little boy in some ways.

He's too big for the little seat on top of the cart now, so I usually help him climb into the big basket, and he holds all the groceries as I put them in. Like usual we started right by the car. I parked next to the cart corral and helped CJ get into the cart. He rode across the parking lot and then into the store. We began in the produce section and got his favorite

Red Delicious apples, plus a bunch of other items. As I walked toward the milk and dairy area, CJ was talking nonstop and somehow convinced me to buy the ingredients to make chocolate chip cookies that night.

OK, U-turn to the baking aisle. When I have a relaxed evening, I might bake cookies from scratch, but not tonight. We would just get one of those easy-bake mixes where you add water, butter, and oil and throw it in the oven. I parked the shopping cart and walked a little ways down the aisle to figure out which package to buy. There sure are a bunch of different brands and varieties of cookie mixes!

All of a sudden, I heard an older man yell out, "Be careful, son!" I turned around and saw CJ had climbed most of the way out of the shopping cart. He had one hand on the upper shelf of the cookie mix displays, and his other hand was reaching to grab a box of double-chocolate chunk off the top shelf. One foot was on the edge of the shopping cart basket, and the other was kind of sticking out awkwardly into the air to balance himself.

And just like that, *crash!* The shopping cart slid from underneath CJ and outward across the aisle. CJ tumbled off the top shelf of groceries and onto the floor. I ran to him and he just lay there, unconscious and surrounded by boxes of cookie mixes that had tumbled along with him.

My adrenaline kicked in and I yelled to the older man, who saw everything, "Call 911!" I was holding CJ and touching his face. Then his eyes flickered open, and he looked up at me in kind of a dazed state. I went to pick him up and hug him, but a woman grabbed me and stopped me. At this point a small crowd had gathered. The woman explained that she was a pediatric nurse, and she was very firm. "Don't move him!" she said. "He might have a broken neck. You need the paramedics here to get him moved safely to a hospital."

To be honest I wasn't even thinking about going to the hospital. CJ got hurt all the time, and once he opened his eyes, I just assumed this was another round. But the nurse explained to me that CJ probably had a concussion; that was why he was knocked unconscious. And he might have a broken neck or spinal cord—not likely, but possible. If that was the case, we needed to move him very carefully to a hospital in an ambulance to avoid further injury.

I had to trust the nurse. What other choice did I have? The paramedics arrived, put CJ carefully on a stretcher, and delivered CJ and me to the hospital. My husband met us there. Turns out the nurse at the supermarket was right. CJ did have a concussion, and it took him over a week to recover. Luckily he didn't have a broken neck or a spinal cord injury.

I guess I learned a few things. First, CJ is too old to ride in shopping carts. That was great when he was little, but it's time to "graduate" to walking with me around the supermarket.

Second, I need to remember to supervise CJ more carefully. I got distracted by all the choices of cookie mixes and took my eyes off him too long. I should've known better. He's always exploring and climbing and reaching like that.

And third, CJ needs to be taught to be careful. I try to do that, but I need to keep trying more. His ADHD gets in the way of his learning safety lessons, and he just needs to hear it over and over again. I need to follow TAMS and shape his behavior.

—Maya, mom of CJ, age six

Maya sure did learn some good lessons, and they are lessons we can all learn from. Parents of children with ADHD need to engage the *act* in TAMS with particular care. They need to provide extra supervision because their children's neurodiversity can lead them to take extra risks. Children with ADHD need your adult judgment and wisdom to keep them safe.

Maya will also need to work to shape CJ's behavior because someday he will need to make safe decisions on his own. Rules about where and how to climb would help, as would efforts to teach him when and how to stop and think before taking risks.

In this particular situation, Maya might have shaped CJ's behavior by engaging him in the cookie mix decision. CJ's dangerous climbing probably grew out of some degree of boredom (sitting in the shopping cart alone) plus his impulsive tendency to grab something he likes (the appealing double-chocolate chunk mix on the top shelf). In reality Maya probably didn't care too much whether they bought the double-chocolate chunk, the oatmeal chocolate chip, or even a box of snickerdoodles. She could have just grabbed anything the family liked and quickly moved on.

But Maya's best decision might have been to discuss the cookie choices with CJ, allowing him some input into the decision. By doing this Maya would have kept CJ safe and capitalized on an opportunity to shape his behavior around decision-making. They could have weighed pros and cons of cost, complexity of making the mix, and flavor preference. Maya could have discussed ways to reach boxes that were out of reach (for example, ask an adult for help), reduced CJ's boredom, and ultimately prevented CJ from the impulsive decision to climb the shelves and experience a concussion.

There's no way around it: parenting a child with ADHD requires patience, creativity, and constant vigilance. Just remember TAMS. As Maya learned, shaping is absolutely critical. Children with ADHD can learn safety lessons just like all other children. They will model your behaviors just like all other children, and they can be shaped into following rules and observing your household culture of safety. You also need to act. Supervision will need to be more intense, and safeguarding the environment is doubly important given your child's tendencies. With patience and thought, you can apply TAMS to keep your child with ADHD safe.

Autism Spectrum Disorder and Developmental Disabilities

The categories of autism spectrum disorder and pervasive developmental disabilities are broad. Some children who fall into these special needs categories have normal or above average intelligence and struggle primarily with social skills. Other children have serious cognitive limitations and may not be able to complete basic self-care tasks, such as bathing and dressing, without help.

Those children with less severe impairments seem to experience injury rates similar to the general population. My advice for parents whose children fall into these categories is rather straightforward: adjust TAMS for the special characteristics of your child and family, but generally follow the broad advice in this book. Your child will get hurt from time to time, just like any child, and you will know how best to sort out the way to teach, act, and shape to create the culture of safety in your household that's best for your child.

My advice for parents whose children have more severe impairments is different. If your child has limited capacity to learn and follow rules, then you may need to change how you teach and shape. Increased action in the form of supervision and safeguarding may be required. Shaping can still be achieved and should be sought, but it may take more-basic forms for longer periods of time.

In all cases, you may struggle with a child who engages in self-injurious behavior. She may hurt herself by banging her head on the wall, pulling hairs from her body, or cutting or scratching her arms and legs. These behaviors are stressful for parents to witness and difficult for parents to stop. TAMS can and will help, but professional input and advice is called for as well.

Learning and Neuropsychological Disabilities

Children who experience difficulty learning in school may have similar difficulty learning relevant safety rules. Fortunately educators have concocted brilliant strategies to help all children learn. You might borrow those strategies to teach your children safety.

We know, for example, that some children learn best by reading, some by listening, and some by doing. Those who learn by doing often struggle the most in school, and they might also struggle to learn your household safety rules if you repeatedly remind them verbally.

A solution might be to remind them by doing. Here's an example from Petra.

Our 10-year-old daughter, Abby, loves to cook. Breakfast omelets, lunch paninis, and beautiful chocolate cakes are quickly becoming some of her specialties. Recently she's been focused on creamy potato soups. Wow, are they delicious!

Abby can handle all parts of the soup recipes without any trouble, but one thing really worries me: the way she peels the potatoes. She'll hold the potato in one hand and then use a really sharp knife to peel the potato skin off, moving the knife down the side of the potato, toward her stomach and chest. I've told her time after time that she needs to be careful, and she should peel the potatoes away from her hand and body. But she won't listen to me. One of these times, she is going to hurt herself! And I'll be the one to rush her to the doctor and then take care of her as she recovers.

After a few weeks of watching this potato-peeling fiasco, I decided I really needed to do something. What should I do? TAMS would guide me to teach. I already did that, though. I was constantly reminding her to peel the potato more safely, and I had told her what to do at least a dozen times. TAMS would also guide me to model safe potato cutting. I admit I don't chop vegetables often, and I can't remember the last time I peeled a potato. But I do model safe cooking behavior while Abby is watching. I've really done that Abby's whole life, in fact. And I've also been shaping pretty well too, I think. I always remind Abby of the rules to follow and praise her when I notice her doing something correctly in the kitchen.

That leaves action. I suppose it is time to take action to prevent Abby from hurting herself while peeling potatoes for her delicious soups. But how do I take action? I know this may sound strange, but I started reflecting on what Abby's teachers tell me during parent-teacher conferences. Abby has a disability in listening comprehension: she doesn't learn very well by listening. I guess I don't think about that much because it seems her learning is really more relevant in school than at home. But perhaps her learning disability was impacting her ability to learn about kitchen safety at home too.

I decided to teach Abby how to peel the potatoes safely at home using the strategies her teachers use at school. Three steps: she watches how to do it; she does it herself under very close supervision (someone holding her hand to do it, for example); and then she does it herself with close but not intense supervision.

I admit that I kind of cheated—I actually glanced on YouTube to get some hints myself, but I didn't tell Abby that! And then the next time Abby cooked her creamy potato soup, I went into the kitchen, got out a cutting board, and showed her how to do it. We cut off the bottom of the potato and then set the flat part we had just created on the cutting board. The peeling was pretty easy from there, and the knife went straight down into the cutting board, away from all body parts. Definitely much safer.

I'm proud of how this played out. I followed the three simple steps I learned from Abby's teachers. I did the first potato myself, and then I gave Abby the knife and cutting board and guided her hand for the first cut or two to make sure she had it figured out. I watched her closely as she did the rest of the potato. She picked it up pretty quickly. I then gave her a third potato and watched her do that one. Yes, she had it down—much safer, easier, and also probably better cooking, as she was throwing away only the peels now, no food waste.

Abby never really thanked me or said much about this new way to peel potatoes, but I feel like a light bulb went off in her head somehow. I think she now understands the safety risks of her old method and the clear benefits of this new method. I never saw her do it the old way again. She learned quickly and changed her behavior.

Upon reflection, I guess her listening comprehension disability did get in the way of her learning. She needed to actually walk through the safe potato-cutting procedure by doing it herself to learn the lesson.

I'm glad I took action, and it may have prevented a serious knife injury. Especially if Abby keeps cooking. And I hope she does because her creamy potato soup is absolutely exquisite!

—Petra, mom of Abby, age 10

Petra's approach with Abby was successful. Each child and each disability may require a different approach, but the parenting lesson here is the same. Be flexible in how you apply TAMS, and capitalize on those areas where your child may benefit and learn the most. With Abby, physically doing the activity in a safe way was the key to successful learning. That required action from Petra.

With other children, you may find modeling to be the most powerful aspect of TAMS. Or you may find teaching through written words is the best way to transmit safety rules, or through illustrated pictographs and drawings. Borrow ideas from your children's schoolteachers like Petra did, or experiment yourself to figure out what works best.

No matter what, praise safe behaviors. This works with just about every child, no matter what ability or disability she may have. When we reward children for behaving well—even just a quick pat on the back or kiss on the cheek—they are likely to do that behavior again. When we criticize or punish frequently, problems can multiply.

Vision and Hearing Disabilities

It probably won't surprise you to learn that children with sensory disabilities such as vision and hearing impairments have higher injury rates than children without those disabilities. If your ability to see or hear is impaired, you may not see or hear risks around you, and that might increase risk of being hurt.

Luckily parents of children with hearing and vision disabilities have plenty of options to reduce the risks. Your child's medical providers may have suggestions for devices or aids to help, but we'll focus here on application of TAMS outside of what your child's doctors might suggest.

To start off, think about your child's abilities and disabilities. Where might your child's disabilities interfere with safety? Can you address those situations through the TAMS method?

Remember also a really critical point, and one that you as a parent surely already know: children with disabilities have plenty of abilities too. What are those abilities? How can you and your child capitalize on those abilities to enable safe behaviors? One strategy I like to recommend to parents is to put yourself in the child's position. This works well for any child, but it's especially useful when you are working to keep a child with a disability safe.

If you had a serious vision impairment, how would you negotiate the hazards in your home? Most likely you would rely on at least three abilities that are not impaired. First, you would rely on your memory. You would learn where things are and walk around your home by remembering safe paths. Second, you would use your sense of touch. You might feel the walls of a hallway, waiting to hit the end before turning. You might reach out for a handrail to descend stairs or glide your hand across a coffee table, searching for the television remote. And third, you'd benefit from your hearing. It's not a coincidence that a disproportionate number of visually impaired adults enter the world of professional music. With impaired vision, they hone and develop their hearing skills. So when a visually impaired individual is disoriented about his location, he might notice the sound of birds chirping outside a window, quickly orienting himself to where the window is and therefore which way to move.

To put yourself in your visually impaired child's situation, think about it this way: do you ever go to use the toilet in the middle of the night? If so, I suspect you may do so without turning on the lights. You kind of know which direction to walk. You might even subconsciously know how many steps to take to get there. You might feel for the edge of a wall, a doorknob, or a bathroom door. You negotiate the walk to the toilet in darkness (and grogginess), just like your visually impaired child negotiates daily life.

By taking the perspective of your disabled child, you can then engage in TAMS to improve safety. When it comes to action, I'll surprise you. I actually suggest *inaction*. Moving furniture could create problems if the furniture's location has been memorized. A new carpet creates a tripping hazard. Leaving a cup of hot coffee or a fragile vase on the coffee table is a mistake when that coffee table might be physically searched for the remote control. Instead leave most everything the way it is in your home.

If you haven't already, you can also take some precautionary action to remove hazards for a child with impaired vision. If the house is set up for able-bodied people, how can it be adjusted to fit the needs of all members of your family? Tablecloths might be pulled, dressers and televisions are at risk of tip-overs, and sharp corners might be bumped. Safety fixes for those situations are simple and quick.

Teaching, modeling, and shaping should occur as well. Again, leverage your child's abilities. Let her feel and touch as you model safe behaviors to teach her to cook, bathe, and exercise safely. Remember that a parent who hovers too much to protect a child with a disability (or any other child, for that matter) may risk preventing that child from developing, learning, and growing. Shape behavior with rules, and guide your child to learn independent, safe behavior within a household culture of safety.

What if your child is not visually impaired but has a hearing disability? Translate this information to your situation. Will your child fail to hear traffic noise when crossing the street? Will he fail to hear warnings from parents, teachers, lifeguards, or police officers? Take his perspective, recognize potential risks, and then take action (or inaction) to minimize those risks.

In considering safety for children with hearing impairments, two situations deserve special mention. First, think carefully about the risks of a house fire (and remember also that most people who use cochlear implants remove their devices while sleeping). Failure to hear a smoke detector can be deadly. Smoke detectors that integrate vibrations and strobe lights are readily available, and careful family plans should be made. Second, take care around water. Warnings from lifeguards or others might be missed. Supervise carefully and teach your child to be aware, using her vision, judgment, and other tools to stay safe in water settings.

Other Physical Disabilities

Physical disabilities take many forms. Some children have chronic conditions that may impact safety but are not visible, such as asthma or diabetes. Others have chronic, lifelong conditions that are highly visible, such as a spinal cord injury requiring use of a wheelchair, or an amputated limb. And still other children have short-term disabilities such as a broken arm or a concussion. In all cases parents should adjust the TAMS method to their family's situation and create a culture of safety that overcomes whatever disabilities are present.

If one word best captures the challenges parents face to keep a child with a physical disability safe, it might be *patience*. There is no absolute, but disabilities tend to slow things down for us parents, as well as for our children. We need to enact TAMS with patience, working to teach, act, model, and shape our children for safety.

To illustrate some of these challenges, let's consider a series of short anecdotes from an array of parents.

My poor little Stevie broke his wrist last night. He was on the playground and somehow slipped off the platform and fell several feet down. The surface below was that rubbery stuff made of recycled tires, but he still managed to break his wristbone. And he's only two years old!

At first I figured it was no big deal. I know bones heal quickly for young children. The doctors put a cast on his arm and gave him all the pain meds he would need. We ate dinner at the hospital while we were waiting, and once we got home from the hospital (took forever there, of course), I gave Stevie a banana to eat and then put him to bed. He fell asleep immediately.

The next morning presented a few surprises, though. The problems started at breakfast time. Usually I put a pile of Cheerios and a sippy cup full of juice on the high-chair tray, and Stevie jumps right in. But with one wrist in a cast, he couldn't pick up the sippy cup using both his hands. He could use his "good" hand to grab the cereal, but he usually prefers double fisting the Cheerios. About two minutes into breakfast and we had our first crying outburst.

The problems continued all day. No use of his hand to play trucks and cars. No tricycle riding—can't steer. Climbing was a challenge, and coloring was complicated. I wasn't going to put him in front of the computer all day. Ack!

—Nan, mom of Stevie, age two

Ava was born with spina bifida, a condition that impacts your spinal cord. She will have to use a wheelchair for the rest of her life, unless some medical miracle happens in the future. We're hopeful for that miracle someday, but we know it's unlikely any time soon. Ava will probably be in a wheelchair at least throughout her childhood.

Ava is six now, and she's gotten pretty good at moving around in her wheelchair. She has no problem at home or at school, and she can handle most of the challenges she faces with ease.

Last month we took a vacation to the beach. We arrived at night and had a nice dinner. We took a swim in the condo's pool that night and planned to go to the beach in the morning. It was just a few blocks' walk. Ava was really excited!

We woke up early the next morning and got all our things together: sunscreen, picnic basket, blanket, towels, beach ball, and so on. We started off to the beach, and Ava led the way. She was so eager to get there, decked out in her brand-new pink bathing suit.

The disaster happened two blocks into our walk. As I said, Ava was leading the way. We could see the ocean in front of us, and she knew exactly where to go. The light changed, and she started her wheelchair across the street. When she went up the ramp on the other side of the street, though, it was too steep. She tipped over backward and hit her head right on the street pavement. There was blood on the road, and I figured she might have cracked her skull or something.

I was so mad. Why don't they build wheelchair ramps that are the right slope for a wheelchair user to actually use? This really wasn't Ava's fault.

I was also mad at myself. Why didn't I watch Ava more carefully as she was crossing the road? I knew she was excited, and I was carrying a load of supplies, but I could have kept up with her if I was thinking about it.

—William, dad of Ava, age six

Well, it's official. Mason is a "three-peat concussion" kid. He's only nine, and he just got his third concussion playing soccer at school. The first one was three years ago, when he fell in the neighbor's yard trying to climb a fence. Second one was last year while ice-skating at a birthday party. And now the soccer game brings us to number three.

This is the worst one yet. He constantly has a headache. House can't be too bright—leave all the lights off. No TV, no phone, no computer. And he's not supposed to "think" either, so no schoolwork for two weeks, according to the doctor. What do I do with an active nine-year-old who can't think, can't run, can't watch TV, can't use a phone, and is constantly in a grumpy mood?

Well, I was trying to find some ideas online, and one blogger recommended cooking. Pretty low impact on the brain, really low risk of repeat concussion, and fills some time. Wouldn't have imagined cooking as entertainment for my active nine-year-old boy, but I figured it was worth a shot.

We decided to try making chocolate fudge. I remembered making it in my own childhood, and I knew it was pretty easy, plus it gives you a really delicious treat at the end.

Mason actually seemed interested. I told him to wash his hands really well at the kitchen sink, and then we started pouring the various ingredients into a saucepan to boil on the stovetop. I left Mason to carefully and slowly stir the pot while I took care of the laundry down the hall.

All of a sudden, I heard a big *thump*. I called out for Mason and got no response. I rushed into the kitchen and found him on the floor. He was lying in a puddle of water, his eyes were fluttering, and he was out of it. Another concussion? From cooking in our own kitchen? This was serious. I called the pediatrician, who told me to take Mason to the hospital immediately.

When we got home that evening, I pieced together what probably happened. Whenever Mason washes his hands, he never bothers to use a towel. He just lets them drip-dry. He did that, and his wet hands just dripped all over the kitchen floor in front of the stovetop. I hadn't noticed because all the lights were turned low. Plus, who would think of dripping-wet hands creating a fall risk to a kid with a concussion?

As Mason was stirring the pot full of chocolate, he was probably pacing and moving back and forth, itching for some exercise and just being Mason. He slipped on the dripped water all over the floor.

I'm sorry to say that Mason's condition was worsened. He didn't go back to school for two months. It was probably the hardest two months of my life.

—Olive, mom of Mason, age nine

My daughter, Zoe, has asthma. She's also an athlete. Unfortunately the two don't always mix. Zoe will play most any sport, but her favorite is lacrosse. Have you ever watched a lacrosse game? Those kids run—a lot!

Seems they are running the entire game. And that's a problem when you have asthma, because your lungs just don't work as well.

One cold November day, Zoe's lacrosse team was playing against their big rival. I was in the stands watching. I knew she was running a lot, but I didn't realize that she had forgotten her inhaler that day. OMG, that was a huge mistake.

About halfway through the second half, Zoe just collapsed on the ground. At first I thought she might have hurt her knee or ankle, but I quickly recognized she was having an asthma attack. Those attacks can be dangerous—even fatal. Coach Jones got to her first. He knew she had asthma and yelled out to the parents on the sidelines, "Anyone have an asthma inhaler?" I sometimes carry one and started digging through my purse, but before I could find one, another mom yelled out, "Yes, here you are!" And she ran right out onto the field to give it to the coach. Turns out it was a mom of a kid on the other team. I'd never met her before, but I sure was grateful.

As soon as Zoe took a puff or two on the inhaler, she was better. But she sat out the rest of the game. We both learned two key lessons. First, always carry an inhaler, and have it ready and easy to access. Second, don't overdo it. Even in a lacrosse game against your big rival, you need to take rests when you have asthma.

—Jackie, mom of Zoe, age 11

Nan, William, Olive, and Jackie each faced a different challenge. Their children had different disabilities and different abilities. In all cases, however, patient and careful application of TAMS would have reduced their child's risk for injury.

In general you can apply TAMS with a child who has a disability the same way as you would for any other child. A few things are slightly different, however. Because their brains are less developed, all children are less able than adults to recognize risk. They may think they can do things safely that they can't actually do. That's especially true when children have a new or temporary disability that causes a change in their ability.

Action is particularly important, therefore, because adults recognize risk better than children. Ava was likely too young to recognize that the slope of the sidewalk ramp was too steep for her wheelchair to climb safely, and William's parental judgment and supervision were required to keep her safe. Similarly Mason's active tendencies plus concussion symptoms created a situation where it might have been unreasonable to expect him to notice or clean the spilled water on the floor. Olive's parental supervision and attention may have led to the action needed to clean the water before Mason slipped on it.

Teaching and shaping can reinforce steps needed for a child with a disability to stay safe. Jackie should teach and shape Zoe to carry and use her asthma inhaler, and to recognize when she needs to take a break from exercise. Stevie was just two years old and facing a temporary disability, but Nan could have used Stevie's broken wrist as an opportunity to model skills such as one-handed eating and one-handed playing, as well as to begin to shape Stevie to develop skills in patience and resourcefulness.

The bottom line is simple: apply TAMS just like you would for any other child, but recognize your child's disability and adapt your TAMS techniques to the situation at hand.

The Influence of Peers

I want to address one other point concerning child safety among children with disabilities. Much as we parents have tremendous influence on our children, influences also come from other people. As children grow older, peers have a correspondingly growing influence on children's behavior. Let's hear from Jason.

My name is Jason, and I'm nine years old. I'm pretty much a normal kid. I love video games, superheroes, and the New York Yankees.

There is one thing that is a little different about me, though. I can't see right. The doctors call it ONH, or optic nerve hypoplasia. I just know that I can't see the world the way everyone else does. I wear glasses and can still see OK, just not quite normal.

One day me and my friends were riding our bikes over to the park to play soccer. They were going real fast. I usually bike kind of slow because it's harder for me to see cars and the road and everything.

I was trying to keep up with them, so I probably was biking faster than normal. All of a sudden, my bike jolted, and the next thing I knew, I was flying over the handlebars. My glasses flew off, and I guess I hit the road pretty hard. I don't really remember that part.

I do remember the ambulance. My mom was there with me, and the ambulance people were watching over me. There were lots of tubes and things all over.

I later found out that I had a serious head injury because my head hit the road first after I flipped over the top of my bike's handlebars. My mom told me that I had hit a pothole in the road, and that caused the accident. I didn't even see the pothole. I guess I was going too fast. I should have biked more slowly. I know the way to the park, and I could have joined the soccer game later, after I got there.

—Jason, age nine

Jason's story illustrates the challenges children with disabilities face. They want to hang with their friends. They want to do everything their friends do. This is understandable, and we parents want this for our children.

But sometimes children with disabilities have to say no. They have to draw a line to keep themselves safe, even when their friends ask them—or urge them—to try something the friends can do safely.

Children with disabilities have to slow down or find another path forward.

Similar to what we saw with Jason's vision impairment, a child with a motor-related disability may not be able to complete physical tasks such as climbing or jumping in the same way his friends do. A child with an intellectual disability may not be able to complete complex tasks such as crossing streets safely. A child with ADHD may need to learn to attend carefully to risks before she jumps into a dangerous situation such as shooting a BB gun or using a pocket knife.

As parents we can teach, model, and shape our children to make the right decisions. This is no different from what we do with all children, but the challenge is amplified when our child has a disability that creates different abilities compared to his peers. Stay consistent in applying TAMS, and incorporate lessons for your child about how a disability may result in changed behavior. With consistent work, your child can enjoy close friendships that transcend abilities and disabilities, and that permit safe play for all children.

Concluding Thoughts

When I was young, there was a teacher who taught us about differences between people by using the basic principle of categories. We were all the same, she explained, because we were all children. We also all had hair and eyes and arms and legs. But we were different in some ways too. Some of us were girls, and some were boys. Some were tall, and others were short. Some had darker skin, and some had lighter skin. Some were talkative, and others quieter.

Even though that lesson was designed for schoolchildren, it applies nicely to thinking about the challenges of raising a child with a disability and keeping that child safe from injuries. Many principles for safety are the same. TAMS applies to children with disabilities just as it does to any other child. Teaching, acting, modeling, and shaping are all critical, and will come together to create your desired household culture of safety.

Other principles are different. Parents must be patient to apply shaping strategies to help a child overcome a disability that restricts learning, remembering, sensing, or following rules. Action may require a longer time commitment when a child is disabled. Modeling becomes harder when you have abilities your child does not.

Stay flexible, and stay positive. Your child can and will learn. Your child will learn to choose safety, and safety will become a part of your family's lifestyle, with patience and persistence. Remember to focus on the positives. Praise your child for successes. And praise yourself when safety prevails. Rely on your child's abilities, and celebrate your child's successes to overcome disability and stay safe.

12

AFTER AN INJURY

I'M ALWAYS HESITANT TO WRITE the common saying "accidents happen." That's because the statement is not entirely true. As we've discussed, there are many ways we can prevent accidents. They don't really just "happen" by fate or chance.

However, injuries do occur. Every child will experience an injury at one point or another. Another common saying states, "Accidents are part of growing up." That one is true. To learn about the world, children explore. To develop strength and balance and coordination, children take risks. If we parents apply TAMS, we can prevent many of those injuries to our children, and we can also prevent some of the most serious ones. But we probably won't prevent them all.

Because we know our children might get hurt, we have to think about what to do after an injury. That's what this chapter is about. How can we parents help our children after they get hurt?

In public health we talk about the distinctions between primary prevention, secondary prevention, and tertiary prevention. Primary prevention is designed to prevent an injury before it happens. That's been our focus in the book thus far. You now know how to apply TAMS for primary prevention.

Tertiary prevention works to improve health once a disease or injury is already present. Imagine a child who suffers a serious spinal cord injury and needs to use a wheelchair. Tertiary prevention might be applied to reduce the risk of pressure sores that occur from sitting in the same position constantly. Similarly, consider a child who suffers a broken arm and must wear a cast for several weeks. Tertiary prevention might be used to soothe itching skin under the cast. Tertiary prevention represents a key part of both parenting and professional public health, but it's not our focus in this book.

Secondary prevention is the focus of this chapter. Secondary prevention involves taking action to prevent an injury from becoming worse. So once an injury occurs, what can a parent do to mitigate its consequences? What can we parents do to reduce the pain, suffering, and disability a child experiences after getting hurt? As you'll see, there's plenty we can do to apply secondary prevention, and TAMS helps us here too.

Applying TAMS After an Injury

It might not surprise you that we can use TAMS for secondary injury prevention just like we do for primary prevention. Acting is foremost in this case, and I'll warn you up front: my advice might challenge you. Taking action after our child gets hurt is tough work.

In many cases the injury will be minor. A kiss and a Band-Aid can fix the situation. After that type of injury, we might grab a quick opportunity to shape and teach safe behavior, and then move on with our lives.

In some other cases, however, injuries are more serious. That's where action gets harder. What should we do then? First and foremost, we must remain calm after our child is injured. This isn't easy. Our precious little one is hurt. There may be tears. There may be scream-ing. There may be pain. There will be emotions. Somehow, through all that, we adults need to stay calm, keep our wits, and make wise decisions. Consider Ally's story:

It was a beautiful spring afternoon, a Saturday in late April. The flowers were in bloom. The sun was shining. One of the first days we could go out in shorts and sandals and be comfortable. The kids were happy, and so was I. It had been a long and dreary winter.

My husband was out for the day with his guy friends, so I decided to take the kids to the playground. I loaded up the diaper bag with supplies, threw in some snacks and water bottles, and got them in the car. I have three sweet kiddos: Jessie is two, Kyla is five, and Max just turned nine.

Watching three kids at the playground is a chore for any parent, but luckily there were lots of other families out that afternoon. I was good. I used TAMS, stayed off my phone, and mainly watched Jessie because she is so young. I also kept a pretty good eye on Kyla. Max is pretty much old enough to take care of himself, but I peeked in on him from time to time too, and I knew there were lots of other parents by the "big-kid" climbing structure, which is where Max was playing.

Everything was great. We were enjoying the sunshine, and I was push-ing Jessie on the baby swings. All of a sudden, I heard a piercing shriek. I recognized the voice right away—it was Max.

I grabbed Jessie off the swing and ran toward the noise. A few other parents were already with him. I pushed my way in through the crowd and grabbed Max. He was bleeding—a lot—from his mouth area. I hugged him and asked what happened, but he couldn't stop crying and shrieking. I grabbed a burp cloth out of the diaper bag and put it around Max's cheek and mouth, but I couldn't figure out exactly where the blood was coming from.

Then one of the other moms shouted, "I found it!" I was confused, but not for long. The mom came toward us, holding a little white object between her fingers. It was Max's tooth!

Apparently Max had tripped while he was running across a little bouncy bridge on the playground. He fell and hit a side pole of the playground structure. Somehow that fall knocked out his tooth, the upper lateral incisor to be precise (I learned that later from the dentist). It was a permanent tooth too—not a baby tooth that would have fallen out soon anyway.

At this point the crowd had grown even bigger, and one of the other moms came up to me and explained that she was a doctor. She told me I needed to get Max to a dentist immediately. No time at all to waste. They could probably reimplant his tooth so he wouldn't lose it, but it had to happen as soon as possible. She told me to put Max's tooth into my own mouth to keep it "fresh." I had to be careful not to swallow it; I just had to hold it along my cheek inside my mouth. Weird. But how could I argue with a friendly doctor when I had a screaming nine-year-old plus two other kids with me?

The doctor was so kind. She offered to drive me and all three kids to the nearest emergency dental clinic. She said we had no time to waste, so I took her up on the offer. Luckily Kyla had found a friend from her kindergarten class. That child's dad offered to keep Kyla for a few hours. Nice.

So Max (who was still in plenty of pain but thankfully stopped screaming), Jessie, and I climbed into the doctor's minivan, me with Max's tooth stuck inside my cheek. The doctor called in advance to tell them we were coming. We drove about 15 minutes and were seen immediately when we arrived. The dentist reimplanted the tooth into Max's mouth and used some wires to make it stay in place.

By that point my husband had met us. It took a bit of time then to fill out all the medical paperwork, reconnect with Kyla, pick up my car from the playground, and get us all home. In the end, that beautiful springtime day turned into a disaster. We had several more dental appointments, but Max's tooth grew back in over time, and lifelong consequences were averted.

As I reflect on the situation, I can't believe how quick it all happened. The other parents were great, and I think I was able to keep my composure

and make smart decisions. I was angry and alarmed and stressed, of
course. But I didn't yell at Max, and I didn't lose my nerves. I listened
to the doctor, managed to take care of all three kids, and avoided Max
having a permanent dental problem. I'm happy about the way I handled
a bad situation.

—Ally, mom of Jessie, age two,
Kyla, age five, and Max, age nine

Ally has good reason to be happy. She faced a challenging situation and handled it beautifully. Other parents chipped in to help too: the type of parenting community we all appreciate.

Let's consider TAMS and break down a few things Ally did well. Most obvious, she acted calmly and decisively. She listened to the doctor's advice and got treatment immediately for the dental injury. That was a critical decision, and one that likely saved Max's tooth.

Ally chose not to use the injury to try to teach Max anything, at least not at first. That was a wise decision also. When a child is in pain and emotions are high, it's not a good time to try to teach our children. This is hard advice to follow. When we're angry and flustered, we want to tell our children what they did wrong. We might want to yell at them in anger or in frustration. Resist those temptations. Treat the injury first, and let your emotions settle. Save the teaching for later.

When the time is right—maybe a few hours or even a few days later—then we can review how the injury happened and what the child might have done differently to avoid it. Teach your child lessons, but only when emotions are stabilized and the immediate situation of pain and chaos has passed. Implement some shaping too, so behavior in the future might be different.

We can also use that calmer moment to review our own behavior and decisions. Should you have done anything differently? Did you apply TAMS successfully? Are there any lessons you can learn yourself for the future?

Very Serious Injuries

Ally faced a serious injury, but Max was clearly going to survive it. Fatal and near-fatal injuries are much rarer, but they can happen. And yes, they can happen to anyone. It's difficult and stressful to admit it, but serious injuries can happen to you and your family. How would you respond? Could you apply TAMS to stay calm and enact the best secondary injury prevention possible? Can you prepare yourself to do so?

Let's imagine your child in a situation where she could possibly die. It's extremely scary to imagine this, I know. Truly frightening, enormously stressful, and very hard to imagine. But bear with me for a moment. Remember that our goal is to help you and your family be prepared, and to avoid tragic situations. This exercise can help, and we'll get through it quickly, I promise.

So hard as it might be, envision your child in a state where she is unconscious, unresponsive, or uncontrollably bleeding. What then? How would you respond? Take a deep breath to consider this unbearable situation briefly. Your child is very seriously hurt. Your emotions are running wild, and for good reason. You are panicked, stressed, angry, upset, and inconsolable.

You might imagine the situation with or without other people. Perhaps you have other children around, perhaps your spouse. Perhaps you're alone. Perhaps you're with strangers.

No matter what the situation and who is there, and despite your rapidly running emotions, you and your child will be served best with calm, composure, and rationality. You collect your wits and call immediately for help. You seek other adults or older children to help.

You call 911 or the poison control center, or you ask someone else trustworthy to do so.

Next, apply first aid. If you don't have basic first aid training, consider obtaining it. Learning CPR and basic emergency first aid is highly valuable and worth anyone's time, but especially so for parents. We won't go into the details you might learn in a course, but a few broad suggestions for urgent emergency treatment in this sort of horrific situation include the following:

- Reestablish breathing and a heartbeat if either have stopped. CPR training should teach you how to do this.
- Do whatever possible to control bleeding by applying pressure to the wound, elevating limbs, or applying tourniquets.
- In the case of head or neck injuries, in most cases you should leave your child still, exactly where she is, until help arrives.
- In the case of overheating, cool the body and provide fluids.
- In the case of extreme cold, provide warmth through layers or body contact with others.

OK, let's jump away from imagining your child in a terrible situation. Take another deep breath and remember we went through that exercise to help you prepare, just in case you encounter such a rare but horrible situation. Thank you for enduring such difficult thoughts.

Now let's hear Vanessa's story to understand and appreciate a parent who responded admirably to her child's very serious, life-threatening situation.

> One cold winter evening, we were driving home after a visit to my in-laws. They live a ways out of town—about a 45-minute drive. My husband was driving the SUV. I was in the passenger seat, and we were both quiet,

reflecting on our good day and listening to the radio. Our 22-month-old, Parker, was snug in his car seat, probably drifting off to sleep.

The first half of the drive is on some winding roads through the foothills of the mountains. Those roads connect over to the interstate. It was a quiet and dark evening, with hardly any traffic on those small, winding roads.

As we were getting close to the interstate, our car suddenly started to slide. Black ice! We were really sliding. My husband completely lost control of the vehicle, and we went over across our lane, into the lane for oncoming traffic, and off the road. I braced myself and felt the SUV flip over upside down at least once, maybe twice. We landed down in a gully. I knew the car must have been banged up pretty bad, and I began to gain my bearings.

My husband spoke first. "We hit ice. I'm hurt," he said. "You OK?" I was spooked, to be sure, but I didn't feel like I was hurt too bad. I took a quick assessment—all the arms and legs moved fine.

"Yes, I'm OK," I responded. "How bad are you hurt?"

"Can't move my arm. I think it's broken," my husband said. "It hurts a lot. Legs hurt too."

"Oh no," I answered, kind of secretly thinking that was bad but not *too* bad. And then my mind turned to Parker. I looked behind my seat toward him. It was really dark, but he was clearly still in his car seat. He seemed to be asleep. But that didn't seem possible. How could he sleep through this? Why wasn't he crying?

I unbuckled my seat belt and tried to open my door. It wouldn't budge. Probably crashed in. My husband was in pain and couldn't move much. I guess I muttered something to my husband—I don't remember—but I know that I kind of jimmied myself over the center console to the back seat where Parker was, and I turned on the car's little overhead light. "Parker!" I exclaimed. He didn't respond.

I kissed his face and said his name gently. No response. At that point I think I was in shock. I shrieked, yelled, cursed, and cried—all at once, I suppose. My husband cluelessly asked what was wrong as he moaned in pain.

My mind was running. *Was Parker dead? What was wrong with him? What could I do?* My emotions were flying, and I briefly panicked.

But then I saw that he was still breathing, and I realized that he felt warm. Good news, I guess. I tried to calm down, but my mind raced still. I yelled angrily at my husband, "What happened to Parker? How did you let this happen?"

My husband was in agony and clearly not in the mood for an argument. He responded in pain, "Maybe a concussion?" *Possible*, I thought. *Hmm*.

Somehow, despite my situation—stuck in the gully below an icy rural road on a cold and dark winter night, car bashed up to the point that I couldn't open my door, 22-month-old son seriously injured and not responding to me, husband in a lot of pain with at least a likely broken arm, and an overwhelming mix of anger, fear, and downright alarm—I began to get my wits about me.

First priority: call 911. Did that. Luckily we drove this road all the time, so I was able to explain in reasonably good detail where we were. It was also lucky that we still had phone service out in this rural location. The 911 operator was professional, calming, and understanding. She told me an ambulance and police car were both on the way. At the operator's suggestion, we turned on the car's brights and flashers to help them locate us. The 911 operator also told me to leave Parker in his car seat and not move him at all. Did that. And she said to leave my husband where he was until help arrived. That one was a little easier, despite the major pain he was in.

Next task: keep Parker warm. I took off my jacket and laid it on him. We also kept the car's heater on. My husband was able to manage that task for me as I stayed in the back seat next to Parker. After a short time, Parker seemed to wake up, at least partially. He was groggy and not making any sense, but it seemed like he was at least half-alert. That was good news. The 911 operator told me to keep an eye on him and be sure his breathing continued. No problem there.

Simultaneous task: could I do anything for my husband? I knew he was not bleeding much, and he seemed to be coherent. No sign of head or brain injury. He was in a lot of pain, though. Not much I could do on that front. We talked a bit and kept the radio on. I just left them both where they were and waited. I was stroking Parker's hand gently. My mind was racing about what all this meant. What was our future? How would they even get us out of the gully? I wasn't sure how far away the road was from us.

It felt like forever, but the police arrived first and then an ambulance soon afterward. They told me I handled everything well. I didn't quite believe them but was grateful anyway.

The paramedics left Parker right in his car seat and took him by ambulance straight to the children's hospital. I went with them. Parker did have a serious head injury, but he recovered. The fact that he was unconscious for at least a few minutes was pretty unusual, the doctors said. He had a serious head injury.

The police delivered my husband to a different hospital. He had a serious fracture in his arm and major bruising on his legs. He recovered too, although he had quite a few weeks at work without use of his arm.

We left our SUV right there in the gully for several days. Eventually we got it towed out. It was totaled—major damage. Insurance covered most of the costs, and we were able to get our luggage and things out of it before it got sent to the junkyard.

What did I learn? I guess I am capable of handling terrible situations. For a second I thought Parker might have died. He sure scared me. But even though my emotions were flying like crazy in all sorts of directions, I managed to get help quickly.

—Vanessa, mom of Parker, age 22 months

Vanessa was right. She handled her difficult situation well. She kept her composure, especially after her initial shock. She sought help quickly and followed the 911 operator's advice to do what she could for secondary injury prevention before the paramedics arrived to take over. Had Vanessa moved Parker out of the car seat to hold him, she might have caused more damage. Had she panicked and delayed calling for help, medical care would have also been delayed.

Vanessa chose to call 911 first, which was the right decision. In fact, that is the right decision in most serious injury situations. There is one exception to that rule. If your child was poisoned but is responsive, still breathing, and has not collapsed, and you are in the United States, then you should call a poison control center (1-800-222-1222) instead. Take a look at the appendix of this book for a list of phone numbers to call in case of emergency in other countries around the world.

Before we move on, let's pause briefly to talk more about poisoning incidents. Child poisoning injuries can be very serious, and treatment for them varies depending on the type of poison ingested. Some poisons call for induced vomiting, but other poison injuries can become considerably worse if the child vomits the poison out. That's because the poison can damage the throat or mouth during the vomiting In those cases, it might be better to have the child do nothing, or drink a lot of water or milk. A poison control center can help you make those decisions calmly, correctly, and quickly.

Concluding Thoughts

What have we learned in this chapter? TAMS can be applied for secondary prevention of an injury—to prevent the injury from causing worse consequences—just as it is applied for primary prevention. In most cases the foremost priority is to act calmly, rationally, and thoughtfully. Our emotions are running wild after our child gets hurt. That's understandable, and it's especially true after a serious injury. With calm, rational, and thoughtful action, we can seek help and take steps to minimize the consequences of the injury.

Teaching and shaping may also occur, but they are generally more effective when postponed until the initial emergency is addressed and overcome. Once pain and emotions are resolved, then you may have a good opportunity to teach your child. Explain to her what she could have done differently to avoid the injuries, and shape her future behavior to stay safe. These steps will keep you focused on the path to a household culture of safety.

Modeling shouldn't be ignored, either. You might reflect yourself on how the injury occurred and your role in it. Should you model safer behavior in the future?

I'll close with one last point. Serious child injuries can and do occur. They are comparatively rare, but you may face this type of situation. My goal is not to scare you. Quite the opposite: I want you to recognize and acknowledge the facts so you can be prepared for an emergency situation just in case you face one. As we learned back in chapter 1, on average a child somewhere in the United States dies of an injury every hour of every day in every year. That's far too many precious young lives being cut short from preventable situations.

Don't let your child be part of that statistic. By applying TAMS and establishing a household culture of safety, you can greatly reduce the risk in your family.

CONCLUSION

You Can Prevent Injuries:
One More Review of TAMS

I sometimes compare parenting to a roller coaster. There are plenty of ups and downs. Occasionally time moves slowly, but most often you are speeding along, really fast, not entirely sure what might appear around the next corner. There are thrills and scares, and plenty of emotional moments.

The challenges of parenting make us stop, think, and reflect. Each day, month, and year that our child grows, we encounter new problems, new tasks, and new opportunities. The beauty and joy of watching a baby grow to a toddler, a toddler to a preschooler, a preschooler to an elementary school student, and so on, are almost indescribable.

To appreciate that growth and change and development, we parents go to great lengths to preserve our children's health. We sympathize with their pain when they get immunization shots, we scramble for Band-Aids when they suffer minor scrapes, and we worry endlessly when they set off on their own to school, summer camp, or overnights.

I'm sure by now you recognize that accidents are not accidental, and that you can take steps to maintain your child's health and prevent accidental injuries. Furthermore, you can accomplish child injury prevention without spending a lot of time, money, or effort. You also now recognize that the TAMS method guides you to raise kids who choose safety, so let's briefly review TAMS.

Teach

Parenting inevitably involves teaching, and that teaching includes lessons about safety. Sometimes those lessons will be purposeful. When we help our toddlers learn to use scissors, we incorporate lessons about keeping our fingers clear from the blades. With older children, the lessons run parallel as we teach them to use saws, steak knives, pocket knives, or power drills.

Other times safety lessons might be incidental. While driving to the supermarket, we might comment about the risks of a helmetless cyclist we see. While walking into the store, we might comment about the young child crossing the parking lot unsupervised, and remind our child that our family holds hands in parking lots. While shopping in that supermarket, we might furtively remark to our own child how crazy it is that the toddler in the shopping cart by the bananas is standing upright in the cart rather than belted into the sitting area. Each of these statements will be matter-of-fact and incidental, but each teaches our child and works to create the culture of safety we desire in our homes.

Act

By now you may have a long list of actions you will take to maintain your child's safety. You know to supervise children where there might be risks, and you know supervision should be undistracted and constant, especially with young children.

You also know you should take action to safeguard your home. Take a look at the following table for a summarized action list to guide you on key safeguarding strategies. Each item on the list represents a quick and easy task you can do to reduce injury risk and create a culture of safety in your home.

Quick and Easy Actions You Can Take Now to Reduce Child Injury Risk in Your Home

Infants	• Remove blankets, stuffed animals, bumpers, and other potential suffocation hazards from the crib. • Restock diaper supplies next to changing area to avoid leaving your infant alone. • Visit car seat check to ensure car seats are installed correctly in your vehicle. • Install smoke detectors and carbon monoxide detectors in your home, and check regularly that they are functioning properly. • Lower your water heater to a temperature that reduces scalding risk.
Toddlers and Preschoolers	• Install stair gates at top and bottom of all stairways. • Install cabinet locks where dangerous items are stored, or move them out of reach. • Place outlet covers on electrical outlets wherever your child may reach them. • Visit car seat check to ensure car seats are installed correctly in your vehicle. • Install smoke detectors and carbon monoxide detectors in your home, and check regularly that they are functioning properly. • Lower your water heater to a temperature that reduces scalding risk.
Elementary School Children	• Visit car seat check to ensure car seats and booster seats are used properly in your vehicle. • Install smoke detectors and carbon monoxide detectors in your home, and check regularly that they are functioning properly. • Lower your water heater to a temperature that reduces scalding risk.

Model

In some ways, modeling safety is the easiest part of the TAMS method. All you have to do is behave in a safe way yourself, and your child will replicate the behavior. But the old adage inevitably emerges, "Easier said than done." There will be times when acting safely is harder, less efficient, more burdensome, or simply uncomfortable. We may not want to don the skiing helmet; we absolutely need to take the phone call while driving; or time is tight, and we really need to cut across the street diagonally to get to the store rather than walking half a block to the intersection to cross.

I don't have an easy answer for these dilemmas. Just remember that your child is watching and learning. That's what modeling is about. There are always valid exceptions, and you as a responsible parent must make the decisions with the recognition that your child is watching and learning.

Shape

Last, we must shape. We've repeatedly preached the challenges of shaping because this sometimes-difficult task pervades our parenting. It involves teaching and modeling, but most important it involves creating, maintaining, and consistently enforcing safety rules. It also requires constant practice. Shaping takes different forms as children grow older, but it never disappears. Safety-related rules form the core of shaping by parents because they allow both children and parents to know what is expected and what is not. Infractions when children break the rules must be addressed, usually by redirecting children to safer activities and very rarely through harsher discipline.

The real key to shaping is positive recognition when children follow the rules correctly. Verbal praise and quick physical contact—pats on the back, high fives, kisses and hugs—represent the true and sometimes-hidden magic of parental shaping. Little motivators give parents incredible influence on their children's behavior, and that power lets us shape children into the safe beings we want them to be.

TAMS in Action: Two Examples

There's one limitation to TAMS that we haven't yet addressed. With most of life's activities, you visibly see the results. You know if your actions yield success or failure because you witness the consequences after you take the action. So if your boss gives you a promotion at work, you see the fruits of your labor through a bigger paycheck. If you succeed in a diet, you celebrate success when you step on the bathroom scale. And if your hometown team wins the ballgame, you celebrate with your fellow fans.

Unfortunately TAMS doesn't really work that way. Your goal is to prevent an injury. If your child doesn't get injured, you won't really know it. The outcome doesn't happen. So you will never fully recognize if you are successful in using TAMS to prevent an injury, because that injury doesn't occur. And if you apply TAMS and your child still gets hurt now and then, that's not a disaster either. The TAMS method reduces your risk, but it doesn't erase it entirely. Nothing can erase all risk of child injury. It's kind of an ugly logic puzzle, but it's the odd reality about accident prevention.

Despite that unfortunate reality, if you apply TAMS and engage in the types of behaviors we discussed in the book, I am confident the risk of child injury in your household will decrease substantially. You will create a culture of safety, and you will reduce the risk of your child experiencing injuries. Let's illustrate this point through Susana's story.

Independence Day, July 4. Red, white, and blue everywhere. My favorite holiday of the year. In our hometown we start the day with a parade: patriotic music, the high school marching band, local veterans carrying Old Glory, the homecoming king and queen in a convertible, and so on. Of course the kids love the candy. It seems just about every float in the parade these days throws candy out toward the kids.

I've taught my children carefully: you can grab the candy, but only if it's on the side of the road. And I do the same thing myself. We stay on the side of the road. That's hard because other kids might run out into the street to grab candy, but my kids know that's not allowed. And guess what? They listen! I guess my work to teach them safety has been effective because this year they stayed and grabbed all the candy they could by the curb, but they didn't run out into the street to grab candy because they knew it was dangerous out there. What more could I ask? A fun parade *and* my kids following the safety rules I taught them.

Each year after the parade we go to the Thompsons' house. The Thompsons are neighbors of ours. They have a swimming pool in their backyard, and we have the all-American July 4 lunch party. Burgers, brats, and hot dogs on the grill; chips, baked beans, and corn on the cob for side dishes; and watermelon for dessert. Plenty of cold beers for the parents and lemonade for the kids, when they bother to get out of the swimming pool.

This year, my husband and I chatted in advance about the typical scene at the Thompsons. Since we've been practicing TAMS and working to create a culture of safety, I recognized that the Thompson party was kind of a high-risk situation: tons of kids in the pool without a lifeguard, parents socializing over beer and burgers, holiday atmosphere, loud music playing—just a recipe for trouble. We decided to take turns playing lifeguard so at least one of us would have good attention on the kids in the pool at all times. If it seemed appropriate, we would pass on the duty to other parents, but if not, we would cover it ourselves so it didn't become a big deal. We certainly didn't want to offend the Thompsons, who are so gracious to hold this party for us and the other neighbors every year.

Turns out TAMS worked well. My husband and I acted to supervise the pool well, and several other parents helped out once they learned what we were doing. In fact, about six of us rotated just like lifeguards might do at a public swimming pool. The kids had a great time, and they stayed safe. We adults rarely had to intervene, but occasionally we did remind kids about how to play safely, watch out for the younger ones in the pool, and avoid too much roughhousing in the water.

My family's July 4 celebrations don't end at the Thompsons'. Phase 3 of the celebration moves downtown, where we go see the fireworks over the river. Yup—parade, pool party, and then fireworks. No wonder it's my favorite holiday of the year!

As we were waiting on the riverbank for the fireworks show this year, my kids begged for us to buy those sparkler sticks from the street vendors, the kind you light up and they flicker and spark as you hold and shake them. I'm sure they are pretty safe, but they sure scare mo when placed in the hands of a child. We've never bought them before because I was scared. You've got a stick that's burning, and the kids are holding and shaking it in a crowded environment.

TAMS kicked in. *What should I do?* The kids were begging to try them, and they were growing older, so I trust them more than I used to. I gave my husband that special look, and we kind of silently agreed to try it. After all, TAMS tells us to teach and model safety, not to avoid everything that might possibly be dangerous. If I thought about it logically, our children really were old enough to use those sparklers safely, and we could actually use it as an opportunity to teach and model and shape our household culture.

We bought a pack of the sparklers and a lighter. First things first: I would model safe use myself and teach the children how to do it. I held the sparkler out, the way my children might, and my husband worked the lighter. It lit up. Wow, even gave me a bit of a thrill! I hadn't used one for years, and it really was kind of fun. I was glad we took this step to let the kids try it, even though I was nervous. I kept my wits, though, and showed them how to flicker it around away from anyone, reminding them that the tip was very hot and could hurt someone a lot if you bumped into her. I also showed them how to put it on the sidewalk after you were done and step on it to be sure it was all put out before you threw it in the trash.

Each of the three kids tried it next, one at a time, starting with the oldest. My husband and I continued teaching, but we also worked at shaping, praising them for using the sparklers safely and guiding them to think about what they were doing. No incidents at all—not even any close calls. We had one sparkler left at the end, so it was Dad's turn. I lit his sparkler, and we all laughed as he spun it around, acting goofy but of course staying safe in what he did.

Darkness was falling quickly. We bought ice cream cones for everyone, and then the fireworks show started. It was gorgeous and inspiring, as always. What a way to celebrate Independence Day: parade, swimming party, and fireworks. All with safety in mind.

—Susana, mom of Wes, age 11,
Wendy, age 8, and Wynn, age 6

Wow, lots to think about in Susana's story. She and her husband clearly embraced TAMS to create a culture of safety in their family. They took opportunities to teach their children about road safety at the parade and fire safety with the sparklers. They acted through supervision at the swimming pool and also with the sparklers. They modeled safe behavior throughout the day, and of course they used shaping techniques, for example, when praising their children for using the sparklers in a safe manner. Susana and her husband offer a great example of how parents can quietly, calmly, and subtly introduce safety into their household without taking away from the fun of a holiday celebration.

Susana's story also raises the special circumstances of holidays. When our schedules are a bit different—we are festive, exploring new places and new activities, and away from our normal routines—the risks for injury may increase. Susana and her husband managed those risks magnificently by staying conscious of the safety risks wherever their children went, and by using the TAMS method to negotiate whatever injury precautions they deemed appropriate to keep their children safe. You can do the same. Practice safety and institute TAMS. Your children will stay safe as they engage with the world.

Let's consider one last story, from Lucy:

Life has gotten more hectic since baby Ivy was born four months ago. Our older son, Mike, is three now, and he's always been a handful. I don't mean that in a bad way, but he's just a really boyish boy. He is always active, just always likes to be on the go and move from one activity to another. I guess I'd describe him as a bit wild too. If there's something to be climbed, he will climb it. If there's some small object to be manipulated, he will manipulate it. If there's something to talk about, he will chat your ear off. I guess he gets most of these traits from his dad because my husband is kind of like that too.

So far baby Ivy seems different. It's hard to tell when she's still young, but she sleeps well and feeds well and doesn't cry very often. She's a peaceful little baby girl.

Especially given Mike's lively tendencies, I've been working hard to create a culture of safety in our home. We've done all the right things, I think: stair gates, cabinet locks, smoke detectors, and so on. We make sure Mike wears his shin guards during his peewee soccer practices and a bike helmet when he takes his tricycle on the neighborhood sidewalks. Just before Ivy was born, I took my minivan into the fire station so they could make sure both car seats were installed correctly. I'm thinking about safety all the time, and I think my husband is too.

Last night challenged me, though. My in-laws are visiting from out of town, and they insisted on taking us out to a restaurant for dinner. Not just the adults—the whole family. Normally I would really enjoy a night out to eat, even with the kids along, but really? A kind-of-wild three-year-old, a four-month-old baby, and the in-laws, all at a restaurant together? I wanted to pull my hair out.

I did convince them to go to an early dinner, at 5:00 PM. I figured the restaurant would be less crowded, so if we had a crying spell from the little one or a temper tantrum from the older one, we could contain the noise and wouldn't annoy too many other diners. The in-laws also were OK with a family restaurant, not one of those upscale fine dining places in town. That helped.

About 4:45 PM we piled into the minivan. I prepared well: toy bag for Mike and stocked diaper bag for Ivy. I buckled them into the car seats properly, just like the firefighters taught me. Ivy fell asleep during the drive—yeah! So far, so good.

We got to the restaurant, and I was glad when they seated us in a quiet corner. Unfortunately Ivy woke up when we moved her from the car into the restaurant, but that's OK. The restaurant gave Mike a little coloring book and crayons, and that kept him busy for a little while. His grandma was looking at it with him. I quickly chose my meal from the menu and started feeding Ivy. So far, still so good!

Drinks arrived, then appetizers. Mike gobbled down some chicken fingers—probably too much of an appetizer and he'd never eat his main course meal. Oh well, I couldn't worry about everything. *But* I did need to worry about some things. I looked up from Ivy and her feeding, and I saw that Mike was holding a steak knife. And trying to cut his own chicken fingers! What happened? I thought his grandma was watching him, but she was busy talking to the rest of the family now. Why was the knife even within reach of Mike? Whoops.

I stayed calm. TAMS told me to teach, act, and shape. "Mike," I said, "a boy your age shouldn't use sharp knives like that yet. Let's see what's in your toy bag." I was glad I had brought that bag of toys along with me. I quietly took the knife away from Mike and put it out of reach. I handed Mike the toy bag and let him choose what he wanted to play with. Perfect—he was in control to choose an activity he liked, the knife was out of reach, and all was good. I knew he wasn't too hungry anymore; he was really just playing with the chicken fingers now. So I moved his plate away too. Hopefully he would eat some of his main meal, but for now he was engaged in a toy we had brought along.

After a few minutes, I could see that Mike was getting restless. Ivy seemed alert too. I was hoping she might doze off, but no such luck. And just as I was plotting how to interrupt the adult conversation to get some help with one of the kids, the waitress arrived with our food. What timing!

And what risks! Grandpa had a plate of fajitas, still sizzling hot. Grandma had hot soup and some sort of fish. My husband and I went for pasta dishes. And Mike had the kids' meal of cheeseburger, fries, and baby carrots. That worked.

Mike was fascinated by the sizzling fajitas. He had probably never seen anything like that. He stood up and went to reach for them across the table to see what it was. That's my little boy: curious, bold, and always ready to explore. My husband saw what was happening and intervened, following TAMS to guide Mike to eat his fries and explaining what Grandpa had on his plate. My hubby was smart about it too; he told Mike that he could try Grandpa's fajitas once they cooled down.

But neither of us thought about the temperature of Mike's food. Another whoops. Mike took a bite into a French fry and screamed—hot! Should have thought about that one. Grandma helped out this time; she blew on Mike's fries and helped him start eating. Good modeling and teaching, Grandma. I was hungry but had to focus on Ivy. I gave her a toy rattle and tried to sneak in a few bites while she sat on my lap. I was careful to keep all the hot foods away from her reach too.

Suddenly I heard Mike coughing. That was odd. I looked up and realized he was choking! My hands were full with Ivy, and Grandma was at a loss, but my husband didn't mess around. He jumped up and grabbed Mike from over the table, slapped him on the back once or twice, and out popped a baby carrot.

Horrors! I can't believe it, but none of us processed the fact that this family restaurant had served raw baby carrots to a three-year-old. We don't really eat carrots much at home, so I'm not accustomed to thinking about it, but of course I have read that raw vegetables like that are a choking hazard and must be cut into small pieces for young children. My husband knew it too, I'm sure. A third whoops at one dinner. Ugh. I knew this might be a tough evening.

Well, in the end Mike was shaken up, but he was fine. Grandma immediately cut all his carrots into small pieces. Then Ivy started crying. I'm sure all the commotion got to her, plus she was probably tired. My husband and I exchanged looks. He volunteered to take Ivy out in the parking lot to get her asleep. I was thankful. I quickly gobbled down some food, and I watched Mike. To my surprise, he was eating more. I actually enjoyed my meal too. It brought back good memories of dinners out to eat in the "pre-kid" era. Grandpa gave Mike some fajitas to taste, as promised, and Mike told stories about his peewee soccer team to his grandparents.

As Shakespeare wrote, "All's well that ends well." My husband came back with Ivy asleep in the stroller. I took Mike outside to run off some steam in the grassy strip by the restaurant parking lot while the others finished their meals. And yes, we had done it! A couple of major whoopses—especially scary with the carrots—but we pulled off a family meal at a restaurant together.

—Lucy, mom of Mike, age three, and Ivy, age four months

Lucy's story offers a few pieces of advice for us. On the positive side, she implemented TAMS well. She redirected Mike under tough circumstances to safe activities. She avoided temper tantrums and also kept baby Ivy content, happy, and fed. Of course, she also made a few mistakes: her threesome of whoopses. In each case, Lucy and the other adults handled teaching, modeling, and shaping well. But Lucy, as well as her husband and in-laws, failed to anticipate potential problems and then act to remove them. In each case, a hazard was present: the sharp knife, the hot food, and the uncut carrots. Each would have been very easy to act on to preserve safety.

In a new setting such as a restaurant, foreseeing potential safety risks and acting upon them immediately are critical. Anticipating injury by identifying hazards is not easy, especially when we're distracted by conversation, babies, good food, and any number of other things, but as you develop a safety culture, you will become accustomed to quick scans to remove risks. In fact, it seems doubtful that Lucy will make the same mistakes again. Lessons learned.

Enjoy Life, Stay Healthy
and Injury-Free in Your Family

Over the course of my career, I have written hundreds of scholarly research articles on the topic of child safety and injury prevention. I have delivered countless lectures to audiences around the world, and I have conducted interviews with hundreds of journalists, seeking to share our research findings so we can work together to prevent injuries.

Often when I travel to deliver lectures, I take walks. I especially enjoy exploring neighborhoods near my hotel, whether it is in Tokyo, Toronto, Wellington, Changsha, or Kansas City. During these walks all around the world, I recognize the commonalities of society. I've visited nearly 100 nations at this point, and everywhere I go there are parks and playgrounds. At those playgrounds there are children at play. In each and every culture, those children are gleeful. In their youthful innocence, they enjoy life.

Everywhere I travel, I also see schools, where children learn to read, write, compute, and think. And in every culture, I see dedicated professionals: teachers, police officers, doctors, and others who help children grow in a safe and healthy environment.

As I reflect on these sights around the world and merge them with my professional interests in child safety, an inevitability arises. To raise happy children, we strive to keep our children healthy. To keep our children healthy, we must reduce accidental injuries. Remember the opening paragraphs of this book: injuries are the leading cause of child death in the United States and much of the world. We can and must work together to keep our precious children healthy and injury-free.

The steps to your own children's healthy, injury-free childhood are within your control. By implementing TAMS, you will create a culture of safety in your household. You will raise children who choose safety, and ultimately that culture of safety will lead to health and happiness for you and your family. Best wishes always, and stay safe!

APPENDIX

Emergency Numbers

---

911   For urgent emergencies in most of the United States, Canada, Mexico, the Philippines, and the Caribbean region

999   For urgent emergencies in most of the United Kingdom and Ireland, and much of the Middle East and English-speaking Africa

112   For urgent emergencies in much of Europe and from cell phones in Australia

111   For urgent emergencies in New Zealand

000   For urgent emergencies from any telephone in Australia

1-800-222-1222   For a poison control center in the United States

INDEX